BORN TO WALK

Myofascial Efficiency and the Body in Movement

Second Edition

JAMES EARLS

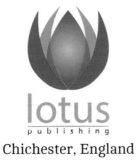

lotus
publishing

Chichester, England

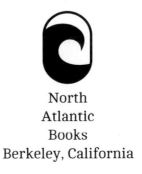

North
Atlantic
Books
Berkeley, California

First published in 2014. This second edition published in 2020 by
Lotus Publishing
Apple Tree Cottage, Inlands Road, Nutbourne, Chichester, PO18 8RJ and
North Atlantic Books
Berkeley, California

Drawings Amanda Williams and Medlar Publishing Solutions Pvt Ltd.
Text Design Medlar Publishing Solutions Pvt Ltd., India
Cover Design Paula Morrison, Jim Wilkie
Printed and Bound in India by Replika Press

Born to Walk: Myofascial Efficiency and the Body in Movement, Second Edition is sponsored by the Society for the Study of Native Arts and Sciences, a nonprofit educational corporation whose goals are to develop an educational and cross-cultural perspective linking various scientific, social, and artistic fields; to nurture a holistic view of arts, sciences, humanities, and healing; and to publish and distribute literature on the relationship of mind, body, and nature.

North Atlantic Books' publications are available through most bookstores. For further information, visit our website at www.northatlanticbooks.com or call 800-733-3000.

British Library Cataloguing-in-Publication Data
A CIP record for this book is available from the British Library
ISBN 978 1 913088 10 1 (Lotus Publishing)
ISBN 978 1 62317 443 9 (North Atlantic Books)

Library in Congress Cataloguing-in-Publication Data
Names: Earls, James, author.
Title: Born to walk : myofascial efficiency and the body in movement /
    James Earls.
Description: Second Edition. | Berkeley : North Atlantic Books, 2020. |
    First edition published 2014. | Includes bibliographical references
    and index.
Identifiers: LCCN 2019048298 (print) | LCCN 2019048299 (ebook) |
    ISBN 9781623174439 (Paperback) | ISBN 9781623174446 (eBook)
Subjects: LCSH: Walking--Physiological aspects. | Fitness walking.
Classification: LCC RA781.65 .E27 2020 (print) | LCC RA781.65 (ebook) |
    DDC 613.7/17--dc23
LC record available at https://lccn.loc.gov/2019048298
LC ebook record available at https://lccn.loc.gov/2019048299

CONTENTS

FOREWORD

It is a great pleasure to introduce readers to incisive ideas. James Earls is a critical thinker; when he applies his brain to a question like gait, the result is worth the effort to read and understand. This is true of *Born to Walk*, where human plantigrade posture and bipedal gait are given the full circle of his imaginative but no-nonsense treatment.

It is also a great personal pleasure, of course, to see the ideas of *Anatomy Trains*, first published in 1997, taken up and expanded into this bold new work. The application of the Anatomy Trains myofascial meridian lines in the dynamics of gait (rather than the compensatory patterns of posture, as it was originally put into practice) is an exciting new direction for the Anatomy Trains model.

We live in a dynamic era, poised atop two crucial turning points. One is the dynamic between the "old" anatomy—the reductive anatomy of the musculoskeletal system as we have understood it since Vesalius—and the more "holistic" vision implied by the Anatomy Trains model, fractal mathematics, systems theory, and a host of recent research on myofascial force transmission. The attempt in *Anatomy Trains*, and certainly the attempt here in this book, is to bend these two ends and make them meet.

"Particulate" anatomy—"this muscle goes from origin to insertion and thus performs this set of actions"—is clearly inadequate to explain what is going on during daily coordinated movement. On the other hand, the holistic premise—"everything is connected to everything else"—while true, leaves the questioner in a vacuous world where everything is possible. So how do we strategize? How do we decide where to go and what to do next and when we are finished?

The "parts" view and the holistic view must be married, and *Born to Walk* gets them at least affianced, if not all the way down the aisle. The physiotherapist will find much in this book to get his or her teeth into in terms of specifics and isolating tests for determining the site of malfunction, and the model is built on classic gait theory. The holistic practitioner will likewise find much to fill in the "everything's connected" trope with practical advice as to how to see, assess, and work with the whole person in motion.

The second turning point we are at, in this early part of the twenty-first century, is the increasing amount of somatic alienation and "sensori-motor amnesia" that we see in our texting young, our sedentary workers, and our debilitated elderly. Clearly, we need an integrated approach to "KQ" (Kinesthetic Intelligence, Movement Literacy) for our urbanized populace—a group that includes more than just city dwellers. I live in a town of six hundred souls in a lovely, rural part of the United States, but I still live an entirely "urbanized" life.

Aside from educating current and upcoming generations, we need to educate our professional brethren. The emerging field of "Spatial Medicine"—changing the body position or movement to change the person—will bring together orthopedic doctors, physiatrists, physiotherapists, osteopaths, chiropractors, personal trainers, Pilates and yoga teachers, bodyworkers and manual therapists of all stripes, and somatic educators like Alexander Technique teachers and Feldenkrais practitioners. In my experience, each of us has something to learn from all these approaches, each of which have something to offer the whole field, and each separate school of thought has much to learn from the other parts of the field.

Over the next generation, all these tender "shoots" will eventually bind into a strong

and comprehensive theory of anthropological development, biomechanics, physical education, rehabilitation, and skill maintenance that will promote a functional body, no matter what one's individual circumstances are. As we move behind the tail of the Industrial Revolution and enter the mouth of the Electronic Era, this effort—to reach out, understand the value in other approaches, and to apply the results toward a grand theory—will take on greater and greater significance, as our children's connection with nature is curtailed and "virtual reality" becomes less virtual and more palpably real.

Born to Walk is a vital step along this path, the bringing together of the holistic and the classical view to understand the uniqueness of human gait in terms that are both practical and visionary, scientific and poetic, grounded and uplifting.

I enjoy the book you have in your hands, and I expect that you will too.

Thomas Myers
Clarks Cove, Maine
November 11, 2013

PREFACE TO THE SECOND EDITION

It is a privilege and a relief to write a second edition. A privilege because it means that the first one proved itself enough to warrant a rewrite, and a relief because it gives the opportunity to make a few corrections and add numerous updates. The dedicated few of you who read and studied the first edition (thank you!) will notice a number of changes that I consider improvements. Many of these changes have been guided by the feedback, criticism, and suggestions that I've received from you. For those reading this title for the first time (also, thank you!), I hope you find what you are looking for. If not, let me know and I will do my best for the next edition.

It is always a nerve-wracking but exciting time when reading the first reviews of one's work. Among the many positive reviews for the first edition of *Born to Walk*, there was one reviewer who rejected the idea that we need any of the elastic mechanism afforded by the myofascial tissue—essentially the underpinning thesis of the book—because to his mind we walk like an inverted pendulum, a commonly used model of gait. After picking the magazine up from the opposite side of the room I realized that it was not the reviewer's fault for not being fully informed—I must not have stated my case clearly enough and with the correct evidence. For that reason, I have expanded on some of the background science to support the overall theory of how the myofascial and skeletal systems cooperate to provide movement efficiency. If you still cling to the inverted pendulum model, please swing across to page 25 for a quick overview of why it doesn't work.

Another significant change is that the first edition was organized around the Anatomy Trains model of myofascial continuities whereas this one is not. The ways in which we move are much more complex than the Anatomy Trains model suggests; there are nuances within movement that require adjustments to lines and to the Anatomy Trains ideas that get in the way of understanding real movement. There are some undoubted truths in the Anatomy Trains map, but many details have been challenged in the research literature. There are too many limitations to the Anatomy Trains model for it to fully explain the four-dimensional nature of normal movement.

The focus of this text is to explore the many dynamics that help explain the mystery of why we stood up on two legs and what happens within us to make our bipedal locomotion so calorie efficient. To me, the answer lies within the interactions of our anatomy and the forces we are exposed to—gravity, ground reaction force, and momentum. Each of these is a defendable, understandable, and, mostly, measurable dynamic, and I hope the reader will find plenty of evidence for the overall thesis of myofascial efficiency.

INTRODUCTION

Man is a model of the world.

—Leonardo da Vinci c. 1480

Vitruvian Man, Leonardo da Vinci's iconic sketch of the proportions of man, is a powerful symbol that demonstrates the relationship between architecture and anatomy and has been a source of inspiration for artists and architects over the centuries (fig. 0.1). Yet it is also one of the clearest expressions of the reasons for our limitations in the study of anatomy over the last 3,700 years.

We cannot really blame Leonardo, however. The symbol was drawn at a time of human history when we knew no better. In fact, the sketch was probably the epitome of the contemporary thinking of the Renaissance. Da Vinci made concrete and visible the ideal relationships between human anatomy, the divine, and the universe, as described by Vitruvius.

Writing sometime around 20 BCE, Vitruvius was instructed by the emperor Augustus to redesign, reformulate, and reinvigorate the beleaguered Roman Empire. Vitruvius wanted to establish a new format for the design of towns and buildings, and Augustus wanted a "Corpus,"

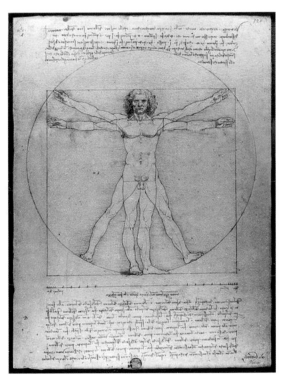

Figure 0.1. Vitruvian Man *by Leonardo da Vinci, c. 1487. Along with the accompanying text, it outlines the ideal human proportions and is sometimes referred to as the "Canon of Proportions" or "Proportions of Man."*

literally a body of work that would encapsulate the reformation of the "body of the empire." Vitruvius's *De architectura libri decem* (*The Ten Books on Architecture*) was the outcome. It was the first work to outline the role and aspiration of an architect, and it sought to define many of the necessary elements of architecture.

Vitruvius's fundamental tenet was that "the power of nature has acted as architect" in biology: universal laws of nature had brought about human anatomy, and so, within our body's design, we had a map of the macrocosm. The body was literally a *minor mundus*, a "mini world," and, thereby, a reflection of the universe. The implication was that the architect should apply the wisdom and proportions of the body's design to architectural design and creation: "No temple can be put together coherently without symmetry and proportions unless it conforms exactly to the principle relating to the members of a well-shaped man."

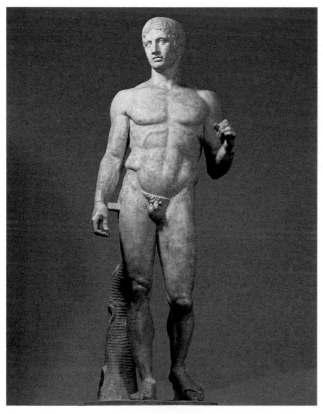

Figure 0.2. *The statue of the spear-bearer by the Greek sculptor Polykleitos was originally created 450–400 BCE. It was referenced as an example of the ideal proportions of a man by many, including Galen, the hugely influential physician, six hundred years later, as well as by Vitruvius and, eventually, by da Vinci.*

In drawing Vitruvian Man, da Vinci wanted to demonstrate his mastery of anatomy and his understanding of the divine, as well as his mechanical and architectural prowess. By encapsulating the human form within the circle and the square, he was demonstrating the divine and earthly relationships of the body, the slight upward shift of the circle allowing the navel to become the geometric center as well as a physiological one (see also fig. 0.2). However, he operated with the tools of the time: a set square and a compass. In doing so, Leonardo set a foundation stone of anatomical misunderstanding within the modern world, by setting out a geometrical perfection of anatomy that would be associated with the tools and methods of fifteenth-century construction.

The use of the human body as the model for architecture lasted for many centuries. The body was used to inspire architecture and the inverse was applied as well, with architecture and the idea of bricks and mortar being used to build an understanding of anatomy. Herein lies the problem with our traditional analysis of anatomy.

We naturally understand the progression of setting one brick on top of another—most of us have been doing that experiment since we first sat up and began playing with blocks. It is one of our first learned constants of the world: the relationship between gravity, inertia, and balance. Just as the body was used to inform architecture, over the centuries our understanding of architecture has been used to inform our experiments with the body. We have walked a two-way street with one discipline informing the other.

Many anatomy books still use the block-type image to portray the human form. It is still a popular depiction within my own profession, structural integration, and was employed by its originator, Dr. Ida Rolf. The language of engineering has entered the anatomical lexicon: we talk about levers, cantilevers, force couples, supports, and attachments. And so we are naturally seduced into seeing anatomy with the same eye that we use to look at the man-made world around us.

While da Vinci may be one source of this misinformed view of the body, he was also the inspiration for a new way of thinking about the body. Late fifteenth-century thinking was dominated by the Bible and by Aristotelian teachings of the natural and religious worlds. The writings of Galen were almost universally accepted without question. Da Vinci was among the first to start breaking this tradition, separating dogma from observable, demonstrable fact. By separating these two elements within Vitruvian Man—the circle (the divine) and the square (the earthly)—he was anticipating the changes that would develop through the world in the following few centuries.

Immersing himself in anatomy and, in the process, revolutionizing its portrayal, da Vinci began to see that many anatomical features were not as had been described by Galen 1,200 years previously. Many of these mistakes were still being taught in universities, and, rather than trust the "wisdom" of his contemporary anatomists, da Vinci undertook many of his own dissections, the sketches of which are now kept as part of the Royal Collection in London.

Da Vinci inspired many scientists to follow in his footsteps. The Belgian anatomist Vesalius (1514–64) took further liberties in challenging the Galenic tradition, and in his dissections at the University of Padua acted as both dissector and lecturer (*ostensor cum sector*). This went against the established practice of having a dissector (*sector*), demonstrator (*ostensor*), and a lecturer (*lector*). The latter's job was primarily to simply regurgitate the writings of Galen as the dissector cut and the demonstrator pointed to the relevant parts, whether or not they matched the descriptions being given.

Shortly after Vesalius's time in Padua, the English physician William Harvey (1578–1657) also wished to branch out, preferring to believe his own observation rather than received wisdom. His persistence—some might say

obstinance—resulted in the medical breakthrough of the understanding of the circulation of blood.

Thus, scientists in the sixteenth and seventeenth centuries began to challenge the orthodoxy, casting a new light of inspection onto many of the ancient scripts that had hitherto been accepted without question. Everything was up for scrutiny, and thinkers like René Descartes and Francis Bacon gave the world the tools it needed for critical analysis, leading us into the Age of Enlightenment (from around 1650).

The explosion in scientific undertakings in the mid- and late seventeenth century included Huygens (mathematics and astronomy), Boyle (chemistry), Wren (architecture and physics), Leibniz (mathematics), Hevelius (astronomy), Leeuwenhoek (microscopy), and two of our heroes for this book—Isaac Newton (1642–1727) and Robert Hooke (1635–1703).

Newton's work on gravity and motion is familiar to many of us. The work of Robert Hooke, Newton's contemporary, is less so, even though it covered many more areas and foresaw much that could not be fully understood at that time. To appreciate the benefits of our bipedal gait and our design as nature intended, we must pay homage to the work of both men. We must understand Newton's principles of motion and our interactions with gravity and the ground, but their roles in gait only fully make sense if we also invoke the elastics of Hooke.

Despite publishing one of the earliest—if not the earliest—close-up images of a flea (fig. 0.3), Robert Hooke only worked with nonorganic elastics and springs, and so we must extrapolate from his work to fully understand gait. But we will see that the interaction between the principles of gravity and elasticity established by these two men, who at times were adversaries, gives a new understanding on how our bodies function. Hooke has been

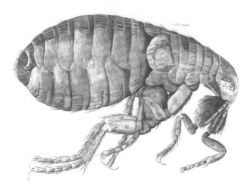

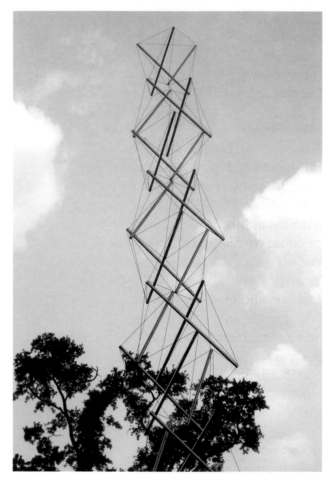

Figure 0.3. *Published in 1665, this image, from* Micrographica *by Robert Hooke, helped to popularize science. It was perhaps the first "popular science" title and included many other firsts, such as the use of the word "cell," as well as early work on fossils, predating Darwin by some two hundred years.*

honored in science by having the symbol representing the elastic sections in the body named after him (see fig. 1.14).

We can unconsciously gain practically free energy through the interaction of gravity and our tissues' response to our momentum. In gait, the body's movement strains the elastic tissues, capturing kinetic energy (the energy of motion), which is momentarily stored as potential energy. As this potential energy is released via the trigger mechanism of toe-off, it is converted back to kinetic energy, assisting with the return movement. It is to this mechanism that much of this book is dedicated; it gives us the gift of relaxed and graceful movement that we recognize through its ease and the flow through and incorporation of the whole body.

Up until the twentieth century, scientists took a predominantly Cartesian approach to the body, concentrating on "parts" and maintaining the image of the body working as an architectural machine. This concept of the body was not really challenged until 1948, when the sculptor Kenneth Snelson produced a series of structures that unintentionally imitated the interaction between the bones and the myofascia of the body (see fig. 0.4). Snelson, then studying with the philosopher and architect Buckminster Fuller, used tensioned

Figure 0.4. *Using tensioned wire and metal struts, self-supporting structures can be created. The integrity of the structure requires the interplay between the compression and tension elements. As Snelson points out, however, while the breaking of one element in a simple structure can lead to its collapse, the challenging of one area in more complex constructions will be less catastrophic (for more, see his website, http://kennethsnelson.net/faq). We will see this again as we look further at the body and how it can adapt to dysfunction in any area.*

wires to support solid, compressional struts. Fuller went on to develop the ideas and geometry of what he came to term *tensegrity* structures, using them as models for elements of the natural world from the atom to humanity to the universe (an interesting echo of the earlier natural philosophers' desire to show the geometry of the microcosm matching the macrocosm).

In Snelson's and Fuller's world, to understand the system, we have to fully comprehend the role of each connecting element. The universal connecting ingredient in our bodies is the fascial tissue, a previously under-appreciated element of our makeup, yet a wondrous multifaceted material that both binds and separates organs, and stabilizes and facilitates the mobility within us.

In the twenty-first century, the fascial system has finally attracted the attention it deserves; this has been due to the groundwork established by many pioneers, including Ida Rolf (1896–1979). I hope that this text can bring a united appreciation of one of humanity's defining characteristics—bipedal gait—by combining an understanding of the fascial system in movement with the principles of Newton and Hooke; the systems of Fuller and Snelson; the anatomy of Myers and Vleeming; and the functional movement of other pioneers such as Jacquelin Perry, Gary Gray, and David Tiberio.

This book aims to show that the body is "designed" along the lines of a different model from that extrapolated from the world of masons, the one so beautifully encapsulated by da Vinci in his Vitruvian Man. My goal is to describe a model that will prove to be far more informative and satisfying—one that allows the whole body to adapt and cooperate with the movement of walking, and that shows how we utilize the energy-saving mechanisms inherent within our anatomy. And, if I can borrow the words from Newton's reply to Hooke's accusation of plagiarism, if there is anything worthwhile in this book, "if I have seen any further," then it is not through my own efforts, but simply because I have had the opportunity to "stand on the shoulders of ye Giants."

And so I must thank all of those who have given of their time to me: Trefor Campbell, without whom this journey would not have started on this path; Thomas Myers, Art Riggs, and David Tiberio, who made the path smoother and less winding through their guidance; my loving partner, Liza Cawthorn, without whom the journey would have been long and lonely, and whose kind supportive guidance and affection made this trek smoother and I would certainly not have reached the end without it (plus a huge thanks from every reader for the many hours of editing—the book would not have made sense without it!); and, of course, my parents, without both of whom the first steps would never have been taken. Thanks to my long-suffering support team at Lotus Publishing, Simon Chiu for his expert technical support, Amanda for her patience (as I often read the map upside down or back to front and we had to double back a few times), Wendy for her clarity in putting the map on the page, and, of course, Jon for letting us go on this saunter together.

Solvitur ambulando, St. Jerome was fond of saying. To solve a problem, walk around.

—Gregory McNamee

People usually consider walking on water or in thin air a miracle. But I think the real miracle is not to walk either on water or in thin air, but to walk on earth. Every day we are engaged in a miracle which we don't even recognize: a blue sky, white clouds, green leaves, the black, curious eyes of a child—our own two eyes. All is a miracle.

—Thich Nhat Hanh

■ HOW TO USE THIS BOOK

Following the introductory chapters where some foundational theory is given, this edition is laid out according to the three main planes of movement (chapters 3–5). These are false but useful constructs that let us build a visual impression and give us time to talk about the implications of tissue fiber direction and force dynamics one plane at a time. The reality is that everything happens in each plane all at the same time—however, it would be almost impossible to write that all down in any form that would make sense.

I recommend that the reader take a quick cursory read through the text once and then loop back for a more detailed study. Because of the temporal overlap of tissue strains in various directions all taking advantage of the many efficiency dynamics within the myofascial tissues, it can be useful to have a loose familiarity with the overall picture before diving into the detail.

Sometimes the way in which muscles are described in standard anatomy texts gets in the way of understanding some of the material presented here, and our initial training can block us from appreciating the reality of movement. During my workshops I often spend time explaining the unacknowledged prejudices that we absorb from standard anatomy texts. Most anatomy texts list the actions of muscles on the basis of open-chain movement alone but do not explicitly state this fact. The reality is that muscles react in the presence of gravity, momentum, and ground reaction forces during normal function. A simple guideline that can often be applied for real-life function is to simply reverse the action listed by the anatomy text to get the actual function of a muscle—its eccentric action. We will see this many times in the text, the easiest example of which being the hip abductors that have to work to control adduction, not to create abduction.

A further problem with standard anatomy texts is that they give the impression that a muscle always creates action across the joints. When external forces are present it is often the other way around—the joints send the force into the tissue, and the tissue responds to control the forces. To aid the visualization of the eccentric dynamic, I have included electromyography (EMG) readings in this edition. If one is stuck in the concentric contraction model the EMG readings can be difficult to follow, as the muscles are "contracting" when they should

be lengthening. We will spend some time in the early chapters exploring why tissue lengthening is useful for overall efficiency during gait, as it delivers pre-tension and strain into the myofascia, capturing kinetic energy that can be recycled and enhancing muscle force output.

The EMG readings are laid out below the gait cycle in order to better present what is happening to the tissues at each phase of gait. In the "born to walk" model of efficient movement, I show that lengthening of the myofascia provides a number of efficiency mechanisms. This leads us to the "essential events," a list of joint ranges of motion that are necessary to effectively load the relevant tissues and are generally interdependent. The loss of any one of these "events" appears to lead to compensation patterns and increases workloads for other tissues.

Familiarity with each of the essential events will give the therapist a list of joints and tissues to check during gait assessment. Appropriate mobilization or strengthening for dysfunctional tissues or joints can then be prescribed to regain as much fluidity as possible.

This essential event model has helped many therapists worldwide and provides principles that can be applied to any long-chain movement. By understanding the movement concepts in this text, the therapist can extrapolate to other realms of sporting, exercise, or acrobatic endeavor. Indeed, the body is not just "born to walk" but is really "born to move."

For beautiful eyes, look for the good in others; for beautiful lips, speak only words of kindness; and for poise, walk with the knowledge that you are never alone.

—Audrey Hepburn

I

THE "WALKING SYSTEM"

Walking while nursing an injured arm
in a cast throws off your balance and
distorts your geometry of the walking
body, creating various tensions and
asymmetries that in themselves create
further pain. My broken arm ached and
it made the rest of my body ache, too.

—Geoffrey Nicholson,
The Lost Art of Walking

Or

The body divides itself into two
units: passenger and locomotor....
The passenger unit is responsible only
for its own postural integrity.

—Jacquelin Perry, *Gait Analysis*

■ INTRODUCTION

We start with two quotes describing very
different views of the body—which one
resonates with you?

The first quote recognizes the body's
interconnected wholeness, while the second
clearly and deliberately divides the body in
two. The clinical separation of the body into its
parts, typified by the second quote, has been
the industry standard until recently. Although
reductionist anatomy has given us a powerful
and useful understanding of the parts, it has
also divorced us from the inner reality of unity
that many of us experience. Interestingly, the
sense of interrelatedness and interdependence
reflected in the first quote comes from the
experience of an author, not a clinician.

Throughout this text, we will stroll either
side of the line between the artist and the
anatomically-informed clinician. It is only by
understanding the parts that we can appreciate
the beauty of the whole; equally, it is only by
valuing wholeness that we can understand the
authentic roles of the parts. Thankfully, the last
couple of decades have provided an improved
vocabulary to weave these two body views
together. From the late 1990s there has been a
rise in awareness of the fascial tissues' roles in
movement, the popularization of the concept
of tensegrity, and a grounded approach to
functional anatomy. Combining the three
elements of fascia, tensegrity, and functional
anatomy empowers a new vision of how the
body might "really" work. Understanding the
terminology and concepts of each strand of
this triad will help us build a new and better
appreciation of the "walking system."

A systems approach is required in order to fully comprehend walking on two legs, which is why we must alternate our vision between narrow and wide and recruit a number of vocabularies to give different filters to those visions. Too often, we have tried to design movement and manual therapy interventions on the basis of either reductionist anatomy or the analogies and imposed aesthetics of how we should walk. The ideas of the correct way to walk are often based on values drawn from cultural, familial, religious, or performance ideals and are rarely based on a true understanding of anatomy. Neither reductionist anatomy nor the notion of movement ideals has provided a truly satisfying model, as each misses the depth of the other and neither appears to have started from the first principle of examining what really happens with the whole body during gait.

The rest of this book is an investigation into what really happens during gait and why. Rather than interpreting from a gravity-free momentum-less anatomy or from imposing an aesthetic of a movement practice, let us start our journey by looking at how the body really moves. Using a range of tools and vocabularies, we can develop a map of what happens, and what happens when, during the gait cycle. We will build a model that appreciates the implications of real-world anatomy along with the new appreciations of the roles of fascial tissues and their connections.

Body Systems

> **New myths are formed beneath each of our steps.**
>
> —Louis Aragon

We often think that walking must be so much easier for our four-legged friends, as they always have at least two points of contact with the ground at any one time. For us, walking requires the ability to have just one foot on the ground and to maintain some form of equilibrium within our tall, straight, and very unstable structures. We walk to move around, to take our head and hands to other places, to achieve needs and desires. This apparently simple action requires a brain and nervous system; it demands internal planning and an ability to predict actions and reactions. It makes use of the many other cooperative senses that we have developed over millions of years. For elegant and efficient walking, each of our "systems"—especially those of sight, balance, and sensation—must be communicating in harmony. This requires the coordination abilities of the brain and nervous system.

One of the inherent problems in the study of anatomy is that we organize anatomy by these "systems." In breaking the organization of the body down into similar tissue types, we tend to focus our attention on just one system at a time. Ideally, we should talk about the "walking system" throughout this book, but, alas, that would make it a much larger tome, and would require knowledge beyond my capabilities. Therefore, I must limit myself to analyzing the body's neuro-myo-fascial-skeletal-vestibular system, and my main focus will be on the myofascial elements and their cooperation.

Homo sapiens developed as generalists; we can adapt to many different situations and compensate for developed weaknesses or disabilities. A glance at the people on any city street will quickly demonstrate various strategies for what we call *walking*. There are many factors—neurological, visceral, emotional, cultural, and structural—that can alter how we walk. The number of possible interactions within those factors would be too large to list and would possibly require consultation with just as many professionals to unravel. It is for that reason that I will concentrate on developing a model of "normal," nonpathological gait.

This book presents a version of what can happen when the whole body is allowed to move together. I hesitate to call it *normal*, but it is a pattern that is inherent within most of us—within the lines and grooves, contours, and forms of our inherited anatomy. It is the relaxed, repetitive walking that allows our brains to be otherwise occupied, facilitating our gift to "walk and talk," to philosophize, to compose, to fall in love, to meander through any number of human preoccupations. It is a gift eulogized by many—from the peripatetic philosophers to Wordsworth and Dickens—and a facility brought about through what Bernstein (the founder of motor-control theory) referred to as *level B functioning*. Walking, according to Bernstein, uses synergy among many different muscles, coordinated without any input from the brain, relying on self-monitoring by the proprioceptive system (Latash 2012). In our exploration of the myofascial system, we will see how the mechanoreceptors are located within the fascial tissue and seem to form a computation system that allows walking to be a subconscious activity.

Your body is built for walking.

—Gary Yanker

I believe the whole body walks. That might sound like a ridiculously obvious thing to say, but many schools of thought exist in the modeling of gait that narrow their gaze to analyzing just one aspect of human motion. As we saw at the beginning of this chapter, one of the most widely accepted theories splits the body into "locomotor" and "passenger" sections—the pelvis and lower limbs versus the head, arms, and trunk (Perry and Burnfield 2010). Another school of thought, put forward by Gracovetsky (2008), suggests that we only require the deep spinal muscles to move. The alternate contraction of the multifidi, he argues, gives us the rotational movement we need to propel ourselves in any direction.

While there is certainly a truth in each of these theories, they are—for me—quite incomplete. We use the whole body to walk: the pelvis and legs are assisted by the trunk and the arms. The whole body helps balance and movement by increasing and decreasing the forces moving through the soft tissue. The whole body also works to lessen the amount of distortion that reaches the head. We need to keep our eyes relatively level, and we certainly do not want the force of impact rattling our brains at each heel strike, so we require the trunk and shoulder girdles to constantly adapt to keep the head steady.

The three elements of the walking system I will focus on most will be the fascial, muscular, and skeletal elements. These combine to form a wonderful, symbiotic map of the forces that travel through the body. The shapes and contours of the bones and their joints create pathways, like dry riverbeds, which, come the flood, will direct the water along preferred paths. The bones and joints assist the body through a controlled pattern of shock absorption, with the folding of joints taking place along predictable lines that send the force of impact into the semifluid streams of myofascial tissue.

The first port of call for our journey through the walking body will be the sequence of events in the bones and joints, in chapter 2. Understanding the natural inclination of the bones and the way they move on impact will allow us to interpret the role of the soft tissues, which—provided the other systems are properly in place—react to the forces by keeping us upright and still moving forward.

The myofascial tissues are not always consciously directed (as most anatomy books say they are) but are often reactive in behavior. For example, the tibialis anterior can be actively contracted to create dorsiflexion and inversion during swing phase to lift the forefoot and avoid trip hazards, but its role changes following heel strike to prevent, control, or slow down plantar flexion and eversion. Its contraction in walking is a response to the lengthening of tissues around it as the foot is planted on the ground—it is a totally unconscious reaction (see fig. 1.1). This reaction is controlled by the mechanoreceptors in the fascia, and thereby we see the role of the nervous system in this already increasingly complicated story.

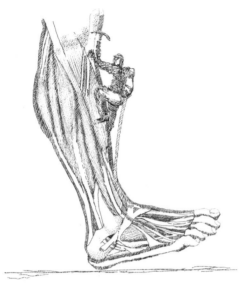

Everywhere is walking distance if you have the time.

—Steven Wright

Figure 1.1. *The impact of the foot on the ground will send forces into the soft tissue along the channels determined by the joints. These changes are felt by the mechanoreceptors, and an automatic response is created by the neuromuscular system to control the movement. Through the gait cycle, the tibialis anterior (and all of the other muscle units) will be constantly adjusting its tension in response to the surrounding events, reacting first to the eversion of the calcaneus and then to the ankle plantar flexion (see chapter 3, for further breakdown).*

The body's many mechanoreceptors are constantly sensing changes in tension and relative position and communicating this information to the appropriate muscles. The wonderful work of Huijing has shown us that the mechanical force at a tendon is not communicated only along the muscle itself but is also dispersed into the surrounding fascia and can therefore be felt by the mechanoreceptors embedded within neighboring muscles (1999a and 1999b, see fig. 1.2). In this way, a change at one end of a muscle can lead to its many neighbors being stimulated, depending on the pattern of movement.

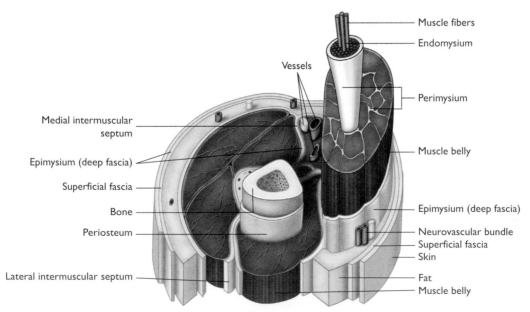

Figure 1.2. *Pull or lengthen the distal attachment of any muscle, and that force will go out into the surrounding fascia to be sensed by the mechanoreceptors. Other myofascial elements can then make appropriate responses to the force in keeping with whatever mechanical information they are receiving from their own four-dimensional environment.*

This means that the fascial tissue of the tibialis anterior, for example, can perceive mechanical information not only from its neighbors—extensors hallucis and digitorum longus, fibularis longus and brevis—but also from the tibialis posterior or any of the other muscles of the leg. It is constantly receiving three-dimensional information of what is happening in the tissue around it and responding to those changes, creating a four-dimensional assessment and reaction to mechanical forces (time being the fourth dimension). The role of the mechanoreceptors is covered more fully in chapter 6.

It is the extra dimension of time that makes any description of walking so complex, as we have to visualize and analyze our adaptations in the three planes (sagittal, frontal, and transverse) as the body moves through time, changing positions. I hope the analysis put forward in this book helps ease some of that burden.

▪ OUR RELATIONSHIP WITH GRAVITY

Stand straight, walk proud, have a little faith.

—Garth Brooks

During my training in structural integration, I would often hear the saying (almost a mantra for some people) that we have to live and align ourselves with gravity, that gravity is both our friend and our enemy. This always made perfect sense to me in terms of static postural assessment, in which we can see the impact of imbalanced segments and the strains that gravity causes.

I believe the statement fully comes to life, however, when we see the body working as the "walking system" of the bones, joint alignment, and the neuromyofascial continuum. Our eyes are naturally drawn to efficient, flowing, graceful movement: the joints moving freely in their designated ranges and directions, and the myofascia receiving the appropriate information, both from the somatic nervous system and from sensing the mechanics of the surrounding tissue. When all of these happen together, we perceive a harmonious relationship, both of the body within itself and of the body with gravity.

It looks easy because it is. Nothing in the body is being taken advantage of, there is no overextension, and there is movement everywhere. The whole body is working as one to achieve its goal. When this happens, we achieve efficient movement. And strangely, it is the inherent instability of our two-legged stance that produces this efficiency.

However, gravity is not the only force acting on the moving body. Once the body begins to move, we also have to consider momentum and ground reaction force. As we will see below, these three forces come with benefits as well as the costs that most of us associate with them. It costs us energy to stay upright, to move forward, and to resist the impact on the substrate at heel strike. Thanks to our unique design we can minimize the energy required for each of these tasks.

▪ ENERGY CONSERVATION

Perhaps walking is best imagined as an "indicator species," to use an ecologist's term. An indicator species signifies the health of an ecosystem, and its endangerment or diminishment can be an early warning sign of systemic trouble. Walking is an indicator species for various kinds of freedom and pleasures: free time, free and alluring space, and unhindered bodies.

—Rebecca Solnit

Evolution and Economy

Walking upright is one of the factors that sets us apart from our nonhuman primate cousins and is considered to be one of the main forces behind our evolution into our current *Homo sapiens* selves. Creating a stable, resilient form with the least calorie usage has been a driving force within nature. Different animals have used different strategies to achieve this equilibrium; evolution is a multifactorial process that cannot be tied down to any one dynamic. Compare the lumbering gait of a rhinoceros to the waddle of the penguin and to the flow of Grace Kelly's dancing. All are the products of millions of years of evolution on different branches of the tree of life. The rhino has sacrificed grace for strength and a tough hide, allowing it to win most fights in the search for calories. The penguin may look comical on land but is bullet-like in the water, where it meets both its prey and its predators.

Homo sapiens gave up strength and speed and instead aimed for efficiency and generalization. Minimizing our calorie expenditure in the search for food—and maximizing the many strategies we can use to catch, find, or grow it—led to what and where we are now. We made use of many factors inherent in our bodies, especially the potential that was unleashed when we became capable of standing, walking, and running on two legs.

Endurance running is often put forward as one of the main drivers for the anatomical changes that led to *Homo sapiens*. While that may be true, and there is certainly a strong argument for it, anthropologist Herman Pontzer points out that we should clarify the difference between efficiency and endurance. In his paper "Economy and Endurance in Human Evolution" (2017), Pontzer defines endurance as the amount of time an individual can sustain a given speed. Being able to maintain a speed over distance is certainly related to efficiency and myofascial economies, but endurance uses other important dynamics as well. Our efficiency is afforded by our upright posture (less energy being used against gravity), long limbs (fewer steps to cover any distance), and the interrelationships between joint ranges (we will explore these as the "essential events" later). Some of the anatomical features necessary for the endurance to run long distances for a long time are muscle volume, fiber type, and heat management (the ability to sweat in order to cool).

During his research into locomotor costs, Pontzer found that changing from walking to running for chimpanzees did not create much increase in energy demand. However, this was not the case for human subjects, who had a significant increase. Walking for humans is an extremely efficient mode of locomotion, and while we can run long distances, doing so is metabolically costly. A reason for the jump in energy use is that the bent-knee, bent-hip strategy of running leaves behind the energy-efficient straight-leg heel strike of walking. In the rest of this text we will explore the interrelated actions between joints during walking, as it is the collective ranges and alignment of these joints—toe, knee, hip and lumbar extension—that allow appropriately oriented and constructed tissues to share the stress and simultaneously load elastic energy for the forward swing of the leg. The swing leg will then heel strike on a relatively stacked pile of bones which only bend slightly (at least enough to stiffen the tissues). Heel striking on a straight leg allows the skeletal system to manage much of the forces and reduces the moment arms at the joints, thereby providing significant energy savings.

Two important phases of gait—the preparation for swing after toe-off and then at heel strike—both require a certain amount of energy. The extended position at toe-off has, hopefully, captured kinetic energy in the many elastic tissues of the front of the body, and the straight-leg heel strike allows much of the impact force to be absorbed through the skeletal system. Few, if any, other mammals are able to combine both of these dynamics because of their quadrupedal stance.

Never run when you can walk.
Never walk when you can stand.
Never stand when you can sit.
Never sit when you can lay down.
Never lay down when you can sleep.
[Especially if you are a dog!]

—Attributed to Capt. Andrew Haldane but adapted from Winston Churchill's "Economy of effort. Never stand up when you sit down, and never sit down when you can lie down." (But I added the last line.)

It is obvious that standing, bipedally or quadrupedally, would require more energy than lying down. Abitbol (1988) showed that the jump in energy use between lying and standing required for humans is significantly less than for our quadrupedal best friend, the dog. Much of the reason for this rests in our joint alignments. When we look at the line-up of animals in fig. 1.3, we see that as weight increases, the limbs tend to straighten. The main reason is simple physics—it costs more energy for animals to walk with bent knees, and those costs will increase exponentially when extra momentum is added through running because of their higher body weight.

Despite being comparatively light according to the line-up in fig. 1.3, we tend to stand and walk with a relatively straight-legged posture. By increasing the "effective mechanical advantage" (i.e., less bend in the limbs; see fig. 1.4) we have created a metabolically efficient mode of stance and locomotion. In his experiment, Abitbol showed that *Homo sapiens* used more energy to stand and move quadrupedally than bipedally, and that dogs had the reverse pattern. When trained to stand and walk bipedally, canines used more energy than when in their natural stance because of the increased bends in the lower limbs required to bring their bodies above their hind paws (see fig. 1.4C). My aim in this text is to identify the many evolutionary mechanisms that gave us an evolutionary advantage by minimizing our energy use during locomotion.

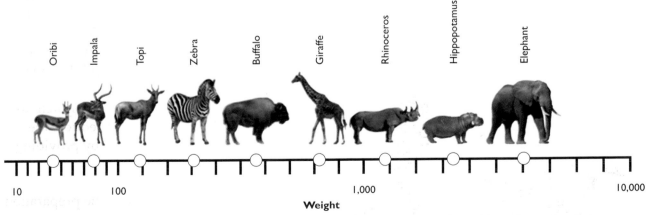

Oribi   Impala   Topi   Zebra   Buffalo   Giraffe   Rhinoceros   Hippopotamus   Elephant

10   100   1,000   10,000

Weight

Figure 1.3. Heavier animals tend to have straighter legs. Increased reaction forces with increased speed during locomotion require more support from the skeletal system, and having a bend in the joints requires more muscle recruitment to stabilize and control the movement. Shortening the levers during gait saves energy by putting less stress onto the soft tissues.

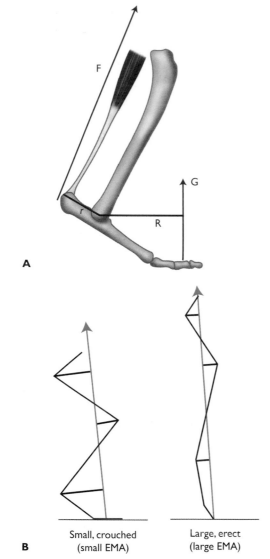

A

B

Small, crouched
(small EMA)

Large, erect
(large EMA)

Figure 1.4. A and B, The number of bends in the limbs and the degree to which they are bent influence the effective mechanical advantage, especially for larger animals. (From Beiwener et al. 2005.)

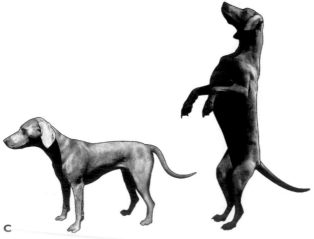

C

Figure 1.4. C, While many quadrupeds can stand and walk bipedally, they do so with increased bends in their joints.

Every twenty minutes on the Appalachian Trail, Katz and I walked farther than the average American walks in a week. For 93 percent of all trips outside the home, for whatever distance or whatever purpose, Americans now get in a car. On average, the total walking of an American these days—that's walking of all types: from car to office, from office to car, around the supermarket and shopping malls—adds up to 1.4 miles a week...That's ridiculous.

—Bill Bryson, *A Walk in the Woods*

Reducing locomotor costs, however, is not necessarily a good thing; although it is good to walk and there are many health benefits to it, the efficiency we have developed has to be put in context with our easier access to calories, which are subsequently harder to "walk off." An evolutionary advantage of efficiency came when calories were harder to come by and energy could be redirected to fuel a larger, more complex brain. Our brain requires sixteen times more energy than the chemical-to-mechanical energy transformers we call *muscles*. With 20 to 25 percent of our daily resources being diverted to the brain, it makes sense that we take measures to ensure the supply of food to this important organ. The current strategy of the average American is to keep bodily exertion to a minimum—for instance, by walking only 350 intermittent yards per day (McCredie 2007). But this is not a good strategy. Strolling short distances, with lots of starting and stopping, takes more muscular effort than sustained walking at a regular pace because of the loss of momentum, which is an important force for the myofascial efficiency mechanisms we explore below.

Efficiency is of vital importance for our survival: if we can minimize our calorie output and maximize our intake, we are more likely to survive. Any variation in our anatomy that will enhance that ratio in our favor will be more likely to be passed on to the next generation—it will be favorably selected. As Cochran and Harpending demonstrate in their entertaining text *The 10,000 Year Explosion*, genetic changes can spread throughout a population surprisingly quickly, with a natural tendency to favor the more effective or positive influences (2010). For example, they argue that the protein dystrophin may have influenced our ratio of muscle to brain, and that the changes in this ratio were selected in a relatively short period of time. Around a hundred thousand years ago, we clearly had more muscle and less brain, but in a relatively short space of time, the amount of energy invested in our brains and that invested in our muscles became more balanced. (Though, as we will see in chapter 4, Neanderthals actually had larger brains than we do today.)

Our nonhuman primate cousins have evolved a variety of movement strategies, including the knuckle walking of gorillas and chimpanzees and the four-limbed tree walking of orangutans. Nearly all of them, however, have to use a variation of the bent-hip/bent-knee posture for movement. This is not because of limitations in the length of the hip or knee flexors but rather is caused by a limitation in the lumbar spine, which does not allow enough extension to bring the pelvis in line with the knees and the feet (see fig. 1.5).

One effect of the upright stance has been to greatly reduce the size of the spinal erectors, which are in almost constant use in the forward-leaning posture of the other hominids (see fig. 1.6). The cost, however, has been to place the lumbars in a more unstable position, prone to spondylolisthesis and scoliosis (Lovejoy, in Vleeming et al. 2007). At first, this may not have been a costly adaptation, as hunter-gatherers may not have lived long enough for these degenerative issues to develop as often as they do today.

Two important skeletal changes in our progression to bipedalism were to bring the ilia

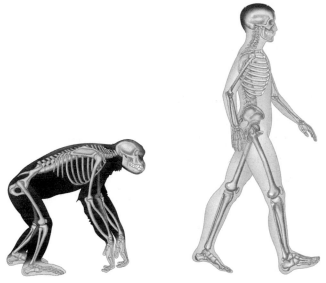

Figure 1.5.   It is the lumbar extension capability of the human that allows the secondary curves of the spine to adapt to an upright stance. This brings the head, thorax, pelvis, knees, and feet into a more vertical alignment.

into a more lateral orientation and to extend the ischial tuberosity for greater leverage for the hamstrings to support upright gait (fig. 1.7). Laterally facing ilia allow the hip abductors to stabilize the pelvis; in other words, the hip abductors stop us from falling sideways when we stand on one leg (remember, we are on one foot during 80 percent of walking). In all other primates, the ilia face posteriorly, and their hip abductors, especially the gluteus maximus and medius, function more as extensors (to push them forward) and give little contribution to

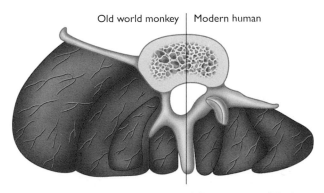

Old world monkey | Modern human

Figure 1.6.   Without the constant need for resistance of flexion, the human spinal erectors have a greatly reduced circumference compared to those of the old-world monkey (note that the illustration here is a "hybrid" of various species). We can also see how the transverse processes of the human spine are more posteriorly placed, allowing greater stability in extension, since they are behind the center of the intervertebral discs.

lateral stability. The lack of lateral stability in nonhuman primates reduces their ability to stand on one leg, an essential part of bipedal gait.

The second change to the pelvis, the projection of the ischial tuberosity, provides an advantageous angle for the hamstrings to prevent flexion when the trunk is upright. By comparing the angles from the ischial tuberosities to the acetabula of the human, Australopithecine, and chimpanzee pelvises in fig. 1.7A, one can see the increased moment for the hamstrings in the human pelvis. Both the Australopithecine and chimpanzee pelvises are closer to vertical; the implication here is that the hamstrings are only brought into a position of mechanical advantage when the pelvis is titled forward, i.e., when assuming a quadrupedal stance.

Many people believe bipedalism was the main mechanism for accelerating our evolution as a race. Much debate exists about what makes us "human"—intelligence, language, cooperation, society, opposable thumbs, and so forth—but the ability to stand upright and move bipedally can be argued to be a precursor to all of them. It freed our hands to manipulate tools and to communicate with gesture. Our comparative muscular weakness and our long period of immaturity in childhood demanded better communication, as well as protection and cooperation in group activities, such as hunting. According to Richard Wrangham (2009), the freedom afforded to our hands through our ability to remain upright allowed us to control fire, giving us the unique ability to cook. The preliminary breakdown of food in cooking increases the availability of calories, as less energy is required during digestion. Therefore, we absorb more fuel from the food we eat, making it easier to feed the resource-demanding brain.

The truth is that there is no one factor that led to us becoming human, but the common factor in most of the theories is that we developed strategies to become more efficient. The changes that occurred within our body

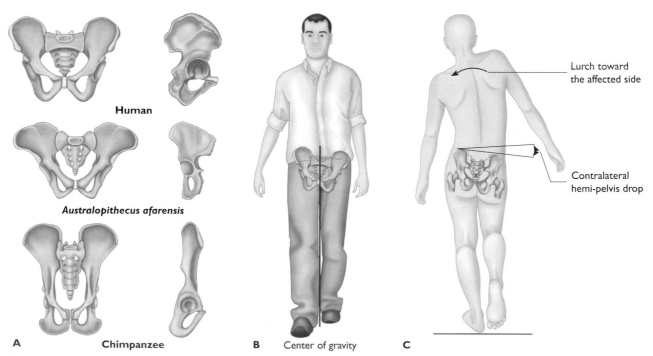

Human

Australopithecus afarensis

A   **Chimpanzee**   **B**   Center of gravity   **C**

Lurch toward the affected side

Contralateral hemi-pelvis drop

Figure 1.7.   *As the ilia of the nonhuman primate face posteriorly (A), the fascicular direction of the hip muscles will be more dominant in the sagittal plane, making them work as extensors of the hip, unlike the laterally oriented human ilia (B). When the gluteal muscles are attached at the side of the body, they are able to support the pelvis in the frontal plane and prevent it from falling to one side. Failure of these muscles demonstrates itself in the Trendelenburg gait (C), in which the pelvis falls significantly to one or both sides.*

mechanics permit a high degree of efficiency, which, as Bramble and Lieberman (2004) have shown, allowed us to become persistence hunters, chasing our prey to death. In addition, we were able to take advantage of our reduced stomach size (due to cooking our food?), our enhanced thermoregulation (we sweat more than other animals), our greater breathing capacity, and, last but not least, our elastic fascial efficiency.

The changes that occurred in our skeletal alignment allowed us to use gravity, momentum, and ground reaction forces to great advantage, giving us a more efficient interaction between our anatomy and the forces around it. We see this when we compare the penguin's waddle to elegant human gait. We do not always recognize the mechanics involved in those differences, though, and this will be

the further focus of this book: the synergetic alignment of joints, forces, and tissue.

Focusing only on the efficiencies of straight-legged stance led to the development of the "inverted pendulum model." This model posits that when we walk, we plant one foot, and the pelvis (the weight of the pendulum) vaults over the top. However, there are a number of problems with this notion, the first and most obvious being that we are not a pendulum turned upside down. That aside, when we compare the forces predicted by the model to those actually experienced during gait (fig. 1.8A) we see that the two do not match: where the model shows force increasing at the top of the curve, the actual forces are in fact decreasing. Now, I am the first to admit that a model does not have to be absolutely accurate, but it does need to reflect reality in order to be

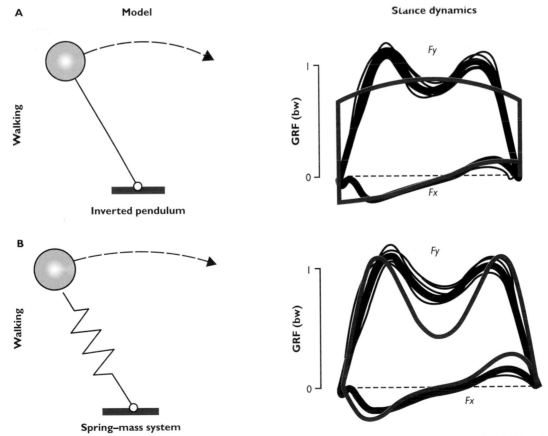

Figure 1.8. The output from the inverted pendulum model (in red, A) does not match the actual dynamics (shown in black), in fact, the reaction forces are increasing in the model as the reaction forces decrease along the upper portion. The spring-mass system (B) shows a much closer relationship between the model and reality. (From Roberts and Azizi 2011.)

useful; when it is the reverse of reality, then its usefulness must be questioned. Thankfully, when the soft tissues are accounted for, such as with the more recent "spring-mass system" (fig. 1.8*A*), we have a model that more accurately reflects movement in the real world.

Springs, Stress, Strain, and Stiffness

> So much of my travelling is done on foot, that if I cherished betting propensities, I should probably be found registered in sporting newspapers under some such title as the Elastic Novice, challenging all eleven stone mankind to competition.
>
> —Charles Dickens,
> "Shy Neighbourhoods"

There are many springs in the "spring-mass system" but only a few, the most obvious example being the Achilles' tendon, have been investigated. The "springs" consist of areas of connective tissues, such as tendons and aponeuroses, where there is an accumulation of collagen fiber. Collagen, especially containing type III fibers, has the ability to lengthen under stress and to recoil in a manner similar to that of elastic bands and springs. We will later explore these important tissues in some detail, but first we must define some of their characteristics and develop a working familiarity with the terminology used to describe the various myofascial mechanisms.

We are all familiar with the reaction of a typical, everyday spring to a load: it will stretch when the load is applied and it will recoil, or spring back, when that load is removed. Fig. 1.9 presents the normal relationship of length with respect to load for a mechanical spring. Along the bottom of the graph, we see the increase in length of the spring, plotted against the increase in load along the vertical axis. In this example there is a linear, or straight-line, relationship between the two

measurements—as load increases so too does the length. Two straight lines are presented in the figure, one higher than the other along the vertical axis and having a steeper gradient, which represents a stiffer spring.

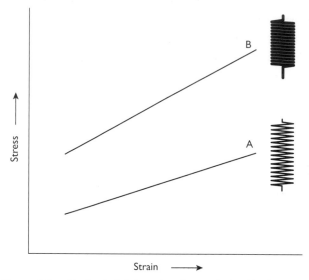

Figure 1.9. *Mechanical springs show linear relationships between stress and strain. The two lines shown represent a less stiff (A) and a stiffer (B) spring. As the force increases along the vertical axis (stress), the springs increase in length (strain) along the horizontal axis. The uppermost spring (B) requires more force to be applied to change its length and is therefore considered to be stiffer.*

Strain represents the change in length of each spring, and both springs shown on the graph increase in length as the strain increases. However, the springs require different amounts of force to change length. The spring represented by the upper line requires more force to achieve the same change in length and is therefore considered to be stiffer. An extreme example would be to compare the spring from inside a pen to that of a car suspension: the car suspension spring is much stiffer.

Stress is defined as the amount of force (measured in Newtons) applied per square meter (Nm^2). It all gets quite heavy on the math, and as most of what we will be exploring has not been measured, it is enough to know that *stress* is the force applied to the tissue that causes the tissue to *strain*, i.e., lengthen.[1]

---

[1]Strain can also shorten tissue, as stress can be in the form of compression and shear as well as tension. However, for our purposes we will be exploring only the dynamic of lengthening

The stress of the tissue is created by the forces acting on it—gravity, ground reaction, and momentum—and each of these three forces will have to be controlled by a fourth force, i.e., muscle contraction. The muscles are not acting on their own since they are encased within a series of collagen-rich envelopes—the myofascia (see fig. 1.13). The elasticity of biological tissues does not follow the simple linear relationship proposed by Robert Hooke when he looked at mechanical, man-made springs (figs. 1.9 and 0.3). In a linear relationship, the change in length (strain) is directly proportional to the load (stress), but biological structures show various types of relationship (see fig. 1.10).

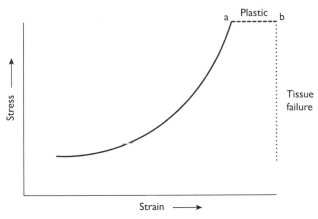

Figure 1.10. *Many biological structures do not follow a linear stress/strain relationship. The curve shown here starts shallow and increases in gradient as the length increases. This means that as the tissue lengthens, it requires more stress to create more change, i.e., it increases in stiffness as it lengthens. At a certain point, the tissue integrity begins to break down and it loses its elasticity to become plastic, deforming without any further increase in stress and is unable to return to its original form. Complete tissue failure will occur when no further length change is possible and tissue integrity is compromised.*

As they lengthen, most fascial tissues will increase in stiffness up to a certain point, after which they begin to fail, either catastrophically by breaking or by losing their elasticity to become plastic.[2] Neither of these events, tissue

failure or plastic change, will concern us here, as they create pathologies and will be better explored in other sources.

Just like the springs in fig. 1.9, the body's springs vary in construction: some have more or less collagen type I or III fibers, while some are thick, short tendons (and hence will be stiffer) and others are long and slender (therefore less stiff). Of course, the various springs are controlled by muscles of different architectures that have their own variations in fast- and slow-twitch fibers. The number of variables therefore creates difficulties in getting true figures for the dynamics involved for each individual tissue, but knowing the general architecture of each tissue does give us some clues about its functional relationships, which we will explore below.

One key feature of the collagenous tissues promoting movement efficiency is its elasticity—its ability to capture energy and return it into the system, just like a weight bouncing on a spring. For a tendon to act elastically, there must be a force acting on it (a stress), and that force must be released at some point to allow the energy captured by the strained tissue to be recovered. The act of stretch and release is the main mechanism we will see repeated throughout the body, once we have more of the mechanics in place.

No tissue can return all of the energy it absorbs during strain, as there is always some lost as heat and friction (see fig. 1.11). Elastic storage capacity of the tissue is known as its *resilience*, and though the figure may differ between tissues and between individuals, the most commonly quoted resilience of tendon tissue is around 93 percent (McNeil Alexander 2002). A return of 93 percent of the energy taken to stretch a tendon is quite efficient and means that only 7 percent of energy is "lost"[3] as

---

under strain. There are many texts willing to confuse you further on the mechanics should you wish to invest in them.

[2] A *plastic* change is one whereby the material can no longer retain its original shape—it has lost its elastic capacity to return to its original length.

---

[3] Energy is never "lost"—it just changes form. In our case, however, it is lost in the sense that it is no longer kinetic energy and therefore not contributing to gait.

heat, friction, or noise (see also the "Fascial Efficiency" section later).

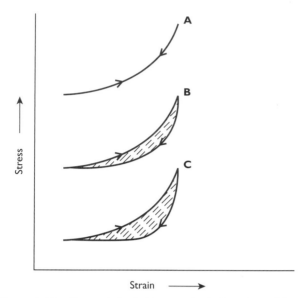

Figure 1.11.   *The strain loaded into an elastic tissue is used for the return to its original length. If the unloading curve matches the loading curve (A), the tissue is perfectly elastic and no energy is lost to the surrounding environment. Biological tissues are more likely to have resistance and produce some heat during movement (B and C), and the difference between the loading and unloading curves represents the energy lost. In this example, much more energy is lost to the environment in C.*

The energy lost due to internal friction or transformed to heat or noise is the result of an effect referred to as *hysteresis* (the gap between the loading and unloading curves in fig. 1.11), and this amount can change for the same tendon depending on the speed of loading and unloading. If the release of strain is delayed, the hysteresis effect is often amplified, such as that observed between fig. 1.11*B* and *C*. Timing and rhythm are therefore important when considering efficiency rates, because if we lose energy contained in the strained fascial tissues, we will have to compensate for that with more concentric contraction from the muscles.

Stiffness-Adjusting System

Stiffness—not the early-morning type of stiffness that increases with age, but rather the tissues' resistance to deformation—is an essential feature of the body's tissues. Each

element, from muscle fiber to tendon to bone, has a different degree of stiffness. While the body's skeletal elements are inherently stiff relative to the soft tissues, this quality does not transfer to the body as a whole because of the fact that each bone interfaces with another on curved and almost frictionless surfaces. One role of the soft tissues is to provide resistance, or stiffness, to the system, to ensure that it does not collapse under the pressure of external forces.

As the stiffness of tendons and bones is relatively fixed,[4] we can only adjust the overall stiffness of the body through active contractions of muscle. As we know, muscle can contract concentrically, eccentrically, and isometrically; i.e., it can pull in, let out, or retain the same degree of stiffness. The effects of shortening and lengthening of muscle fibers occurs via actin and myosin filaments drawing together or spreading apart, which require a greater exchange of metabolic energy and influence the potential for force output (see fig. 1.12). A concentrically shortened or eccentrically lengthened muscle will have lower potential for force output and will have used more metabolic resources by changing length.

To explain the importance of this, we need to look at normal movement. A number of experiments have shown that during repetitive movements such as walking, there is very little change in the length of the muscle fibers, which are often used in isometric contraction (i.e., they are not changing length when they contract—they are simply maintaining their current length; see fig. 1.14). Much of the lengthening required during walking actually occurs in the fascial tissues, in the collagen and elastin, which are able to recoil from the stretch and return to their resting length, like a spring.

The benefits of this arrangement are twofold: the recoil of the fascial tissue provides

---

[4]Tissue stiffness can change over time as a result of physiological changes, such as pathology, ageing, or nutritional effects. The stiffness of muscle tone, on the other hand, adjusts almost instantaneously.

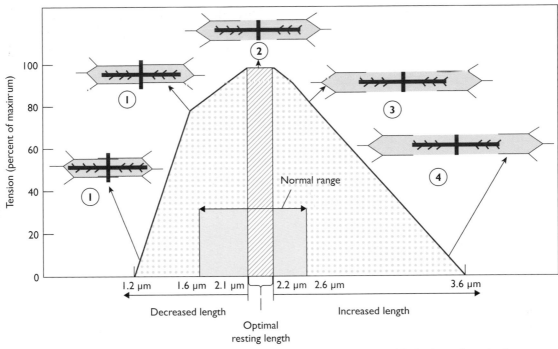

Figure 1.12. *Force–length of a muscle. As a result of actin fibers (in red) and myosin (in dark blue) relationships, the force output is affected by the muscle's length and has an optimal midrange for maximum force output. 1. The actin fibers overlap and reduce the ability of any further shortening. 2. The ideal overlap between actin and myosin fibers. 3 & 4. As the muscle lengthens, fewer myosin filaments overlap with the actin elements thereby reducing the purchase for contraction.*

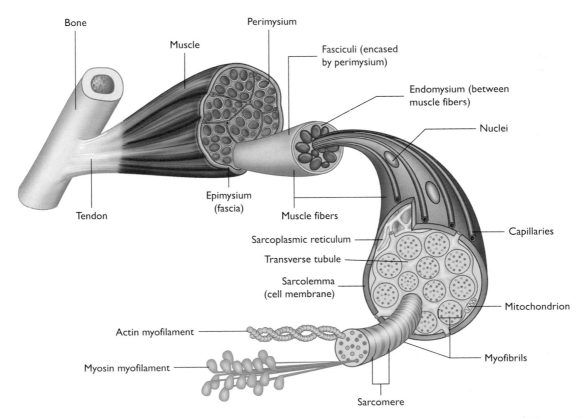

Figure 1.13. *Each muscle is encased within a series of fascial bags—the epimysium, perimysium, and endomysium—which are made up of various types of collagen fiber, with a blend of elastin and the more-fluid ground substance.*

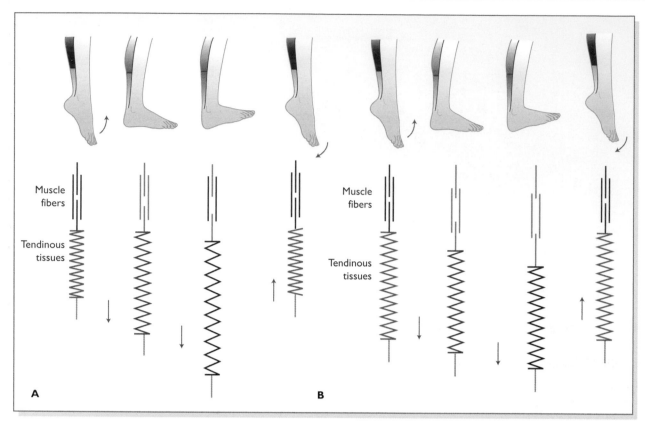

Figure 1.14.   In this diagram, the fascial tissue is represented as the "elastic" tissue (using Hookean springs) and the contractile muscle as sliding filaments. In a series of experiments, Kawakami et al. (2006) showed that in cyclical movements the muscles tended to remain predominantly isometric (A) rather than doing the extra work on concentric and eccentric contraction (B).

essentially free energy, and the muscle can stay within its optimal force–length relationship. Because the muscles remain close to isometric functioning, the force involved in the body's momentum will strain the collagenous tissues. The collagenous tissues transform kinetic energy into potential energy by absorbing energy and then releasing it back into the system as kinetic energy again. By allowing the fascial tissues to lengthen, the muscle does not stray into the metabolically expensive and weaker shortened and lengthened states.

Once again, we see the body's drive for efficiency come into play, but it can only utilize this mechanism when there are sufficient external forces present: momentum and ground reaction forces are necessary in order to create enough strain on the collagenous tissues. The active concentric and eccentric contraction of muscles is expensive, requiring the exchange of adenosine triphosphate (ATP) and glucose, while much less fuel is required when muscle

fibers are held in isometric contraction. The hallmarks of efficient walking are minimizing muscular work and maximizing recoil efficiency of the fascial tissues. If we walk more slowly and lose momentum, however, we have to replace the reduced elasticity with concentric and eccentric contraction.

In exploring the body's drive for efficiency, Sawicki et al. (2009) and Farley et al. (1998) among others discovered indications that a muscle constantly fine-tunes its length in response to changes in forces, and it does this to minimize metabolic cost. For example, Sawicki and colleagues measured muscle work during normal gait and then with a robotic exoskeleton which provided an external spring similar to that of the Achilles's tendon. They found that subjects quickly re-tuned their calf muscles to do less work, and their overall metabolic cost decreased. Their work implies that muscle tissue can sense the assistance it is receiving from external sources and adjust

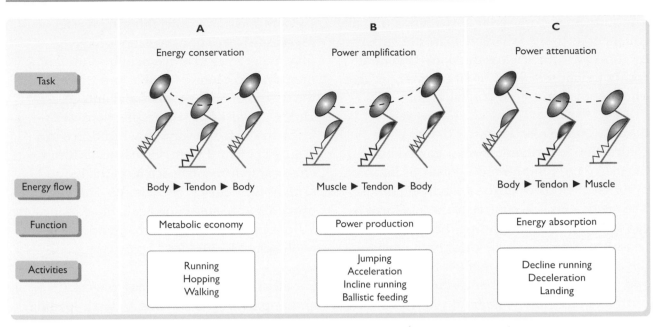

	A	B	C
Task	Energy conservation	Power amplification	Power attenuation
Energy flow	Body ▶ Tendon ▶ Body	Muscle ▶ Tendon ▶ Body	Body ▶ Tendon ▶ Muscle
Function	Metabolic economy	Power production	Energy absorption
Activities	Running / Hopping / Walking	Jumping / Acceleration / Incline running / Ballistic feeding	Decline running / Deceleration / Landing

Figure 1.15. The three main functions of myofascial tissue during movement. (From Roberts and Azizi 2011.)

its tone to maximize the recycling of kinetic energy and to minimize its own work. Muscles, it seems, are a little work-shy.

To avoid changing length, muscles need external stress to strain the collagenous tissues. This tissue strain during movement is created by the stressors of momentum, gravity, and ground reaction forces. Each of those forces must be allowed to travel through the system to spread the load among the body's tissues. In subsequent chapters, we will explore the various channels the forces follow to allow the soft tissues to maintain an optimal force–length relationship.

The mechanism described in the previous few pages is that of energy conservation— the loading and unloading of elastic energy into tendons increases the overall movement efficiency. There are three main roles of the fascial tissue in movement (fig. 1.15): energy conservation, power amplification, and power attenuation (or, damping). Although we will explore power amplification below, it is less relevant to walking, and so only a little time will be spent on this to clarify the attenuation that happens when decelerating or stopping a movement. When the foot lands or you stop during walking, some energy will be absorbed

by the tendon, and the muscle then "lets out" by eccentrically contracting to dissipate the energy in the strained tendon.

Power Amplification

> **Today is one of those excellent January partly cloudies in which light chooses an unexpected part of the landscape to trick out in gilt, and then the shadow sweeps it away. You know you're alive. You take huge steps, trying to feel the planet's roundness arc between your feet.**
>
> —Annie Dillard, *Pilgrim at Tinker Creek*

As we have already seen, when momentum is present, the muscle fiber can retain its optimum force–length relationship. The strain on the collagenous tissues will also have loaded energy, which can then be used for the return movement, helping further reduce the muscle effort. The collagenous tissue will be pre-stiffened by the momentum, meaning that the early stages of strain (seen in fig. 1.10 as the low gradient of the foot of the slope) will have been taken up by the movement. If this low stiffness is not used up by momentum, the collagenous tissue will have to be pre-stiffened by concentric muscle contraction—potentially taking the muscle fiber into its shorter, weaker phase of the force–length relationship.

Because elastic recoil is faster than muscle contraction, a further benefit is gained by the use of the catapult mechanism, as it can optimize the muscle force–velocity relationship. The faster a muscle contracts, the less force it can produce. By first loading the surrounding fascial collagenous tissue prior to the release, the elastic load can create the initial impetus and allow the muscle fiber contained within to contract more slowly, hopefully when its force–velocity ratio is optimal.

The use of elastic recoil and force amplification explains why most of our movements begin with a movement in the opposite direction. A countermovement requires the muscle to decelerate the preparatory movement. The momentum pre-stiffens the tissues and loads extra energy into the fascial tissues, which can then assist with the intended action. The movement requires less muscle contraction because the muscles have been allowed to remain close to isometric; they will contract within a pre-stiffened bag (and not have to "take up the slack" before contraction is felt at either attachment). The fascial "bag" can also contribute some elastic energy, and both the force–length and force–velocity relationships are enhanced.

This description of the dynamic has emphasized the in-series relationships of the myofascial tissues. However, as we will see later, force amplification also occurs in parallel. Our layered tissues can work for one another: as one layer stiffens, it will assist the stiffening of the layers above and below in a mutually beneficial arrangement. As mentioned above, over many years the work of Prof. Huijing has shown how force transmits through the myofascial tissues not only horizontally, along the muscle-tendon unit, but also beyond its

borders and into the neighboring tissues. Myofascial force transmission is likely to play many roles in movement by stimulating mechanoreceptors, as well as pre-stiffening the tissues of both agonists and antagonists.[5] Huijing's work has shown that there are few barriers to the ways in which force can migrate outward from one tissue, as it can cross compartments (such as in the leg and arm) as well muscle borders. We will encounter in-parallel pre-stiffening again on exploring the actions around the hip in chapter 5 and below in "Fascial Membranes."

For all of the above dynamics to work (in-series and in-parallel pre-stiffening, elastic loading, and recoil), countermovement has to occur in the appropriate tissues. If we cannot load with a countermovement, we will have to compensate with some form of concentric contraction to accomplish the desired movement. The countermovement is created by a number of dynamics, the obvious one being momentum; however, the offsets between centers of support and centers of gravity in our skeletal structure (such as in the hip abductors mentioned above) also allow ground reaction force and gravity to play important roles.

■ FORCES AT WORK— GRAVITY AND GROUND REACTION FORCE

When you walk on earth, you must know that one miracle walks on another miracle!

—Mehmet Murat ildan

[5] I hesitate to use the terms *agonist* and *antagonist* as they portray a simplistic binary-type system such as the one I was first taught many years ago. I prefer to see all of the tissues as *agonists* for any movement—they are all helping support the system to produce the desired action; it is just that some might be elongating, some might be shortening, and some might be staying the same length.

"Ground reaction force" may sound like a subterranean terrorist group (fig. 1.16), but it is actually a vitally important aspect of understanding what is happening during gait; unfortunately, it is also probably one of the most confused aspects. This is the stage where many readers may be tempted to skip a few pages, as they feel the imminence of another "science bit", but please hold true for just a few pages. It will serve you very well, not just for the rest of this book, but also in the understanding of any human movement.

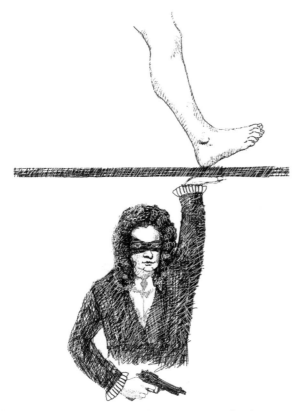

Figure 1.16. *Ground reaction force is more complex than a simple rebounding of energy, as would be predicted from a simple understanding of Newton's third law.*

One of the problems with explaining ground reaction force is that it begins to invoke physics, and everyone loves to quote Newton's third law: "To every action there is an equal and opposite reaction." What this means is that when my foot hits the ground, the ground pushes right back at me with the same force, but in the opposite direction, and this helps keep me upright. Sometimes in movement classes, instructors encourage their students,

"push into the ground and feel it push you back up." Unfortunately, this is a bit of an oversimplification.

Let us begin with the difference between walking on asphalt and walking on sand—we all know the extra work that is needed when sauntering across a beach. Taking the example of the asphalt first: when we push into it, the surface will deform slightly (not enough for us to notice it with ordinary human senses, but it does happen), and it will return to its original state as we push off from it.

When we walk on the beach, however, the force with which we push into the surface is used to displace many thousands of grains of sand. The grains are not connected to one another, and so the beach does not have an elastic capability to regain its original form. When we heel strike in sand, most of the force is therefore dispersed and gets lost in the movement of the grains.

If we looked very closely at the sand, we could see that the movement of each grain will depend on its shape and the angle from which it is pushed. Because the grains of sand are not bonded together, these changes are similar to those when hitting balls on a pool table. Once the force stops acting on the grains (or balls), they come to rest where they are, rather than returning to their starting position.

Much of the energy inherent in the foot strike is used up by the displacement of the sand. Now imagine that the grains of sand were joined to one another by strong elastic bands. Each of those movements by the sand would be reversible, just like the bounce on a trampoline, which is temporarily displaced but, because of the elasticity of its springs, returns to its original shape.

Until now we have considered the body to be a reasonably solid object—when imagining a body jumping on a trampoline, the discussion focused only on the stretching of the trampoline. But actually, the body is also being "displaced"—stretched and moved—when it lands on the trampoline. The skeleton is analogous to the grains of sand, with each bone being moved in a different way through the interaction of gravity, momentum, and ground reaction force. In the human body, however, the bones are held together by elastic tissue, the myofascia, which absorbs the forces coming from each of these three dynamics.

A full exploration of ground reaction force would be much more complicated than we need for our overall picture of the economy and cooperation of walking (and it can sprout lots of scary-looking equations). A simplified version of how ground reaction force works, however, will help us see what happens in the body when it interacts with the ground.

If we look at a skeleton, we can see the bones are offset and stacked on top of one another, with extremely slippery surfaces (see also "Tensegrity" below). The skeleton therefore provides very little inherent stability to our body; instead, each bone acts as a stiff anchor for the stiffness-adjusting myofascia. By virtue of their unstable nature, the bones also assist with the production of pre-stiffening countermovements. The offset of each bone creates an offset between ground reaction force coming up through the body and gravity (with momentum) coming down. The offsetting of the forces causes each bone to tilt, turn, or shift, thereby creating another local countermovement to pre-stiffen the tissues local to the bones. It may seem counterintuitive, but going in the opposite direction (but not too far!) helps with the efficiency of our movement. Countermovement, as you will see, is vital to our understanding of walking, and we must be able to visualize the interactions between the forward momentum of gait, the downward force of gravity, and the upward ground reaction forces.

For example, the interaction between the foot and the ground is relatively simple when one is standing still. In walking, however, the ground

reaction force is not perpendicular to gravity. It is this angle of impact that invokes the folding of the joints throughout the body, and, as we will see as we progress through the book, it is the controlled adjustment of the joints that "loads" the tissue to assist recovery and recoil. (The springs of the trampoline can be seen as an analogy. They are stretched—"loaded" with recoil power—when someone jumps on the trampoline.)

To fully understand ground reaction force, we have to view it in the context of other variables—gravity, momentum, and surface stiffness. Whereas gravity is constant with respect to force and angle (fig. 1.17), the ground reaction force will alter its vector according to the angle at which the surface is struck (fig. 1.18). The ground reaction force received

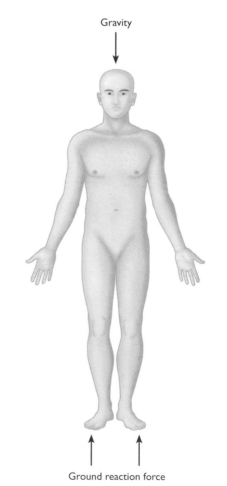

Gravity

Ground reaction force

Figure 1.17. When one is standing quietly, gravity is pulling the center of gravity down, and this is being "met" by the ground reaction force pushing straight up.

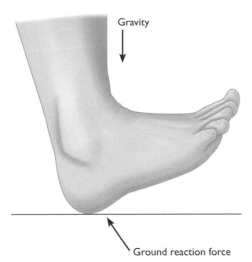

Gravity

Ground reaction force

Figure 1.18. *As the heel hits the floor, the ground reaction force "pushes" back at the heel in the opposite direction; this is what decelerates movement of the calcaneus.*

by the body following impact will depend on the interaction between the momentum and the surface stiffness—a heavy heel strike on sand will be less shocking to the system than the same heel strike on concrete.

■ MYOFASCIAL DESIGN

The eccentric lengthening of the tissue created by the shock absorption also helps the body return in the opposite direction, just like the springs of the trampoline. The myofascia is

mechanically loaded, like springs, through the momentum created by the forward and rotational forces of walking, as well as by the pull of gravity. This is performed through relatively passive mechanisms (rather than through muscle contraction) that allow the elastic fascial tissue to be put under stretch in all three planes of motion. Because of the angles and positions of the joints in the body, these forces are not restricted to single muscles, as demonstrated by the work carried out by Huijing and Vleeming among others.

When the fascial tissue is stretched over joints, it may sometimes transfer force across the joint from one myofascial unit to another. When the joints are in midrange, the associated tissue is less stiff and communication is limited to the single myofascial units on one side of the joint (see exercise 1.1), but in certain stretched positions, closer to the end of range, force transmission may be facilitated along the myofascia across the joints.

Exercise 1.1. **First, extend your wrist and fingers to feel the stretch and then compare the sensation and range of motion when you repeat the wrist extension with your elbow also extended (fig. 1.19). Finally, draw your arm back and into horizontal abduction,**

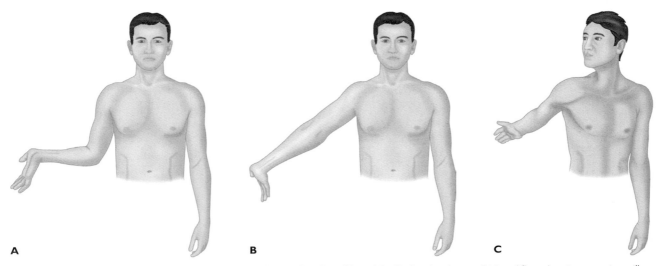

A   B   C

Figure 1.19. *By engaging the tissues across the wrist (A), then the elbow (B), and finally the glenohumeral joints (C), each wrist extension will feel differently as more of the anterior arm tissue is brought into the movement. Experiment further by changing the position and angle of the humerus and noticing the effect on the stretch of the wrist flexors. You may find there is a certain angle and position that feels as if it includes all of the anterior tissue. It is this mechanism—the proper positioning that engages the entire anterior tissue—that we wish to exploit in walking.*

keep your elbow extended, and again extend your wrist. Each of these movements will engage more tissue across each subsequent joint. They may or may not affect the range of motion, but the sensations should differ as you bring into play more tissues because of the joint extensions. As each joint extends, the communication of force across the joints is facilitated and this is an underpinning element of how we walk efficiently—loading elastic energy into passive tissues requires enough movement at each joint to allow force dispersal and distribution. Failure to distribute kinetic energy will cause overuse of the tissues, as they either absorb too much kinetic energy or have to concentrically contract repetitively to create the energy to move.

When longer lines of myofascia are engaged, one part of the body can affect another. Just as the shoulder position affects the hand and wrist in exercise 1.1, so too will the pelvis affect the foot; and likewise, the head, the thorax. By visualizing continuous lines of force through the body, we can interpret the effects of one part on another, understanding how, for example, the shoulder position may affect the tracking of the knee. This will, hopefully, lead to ways of correcting inefficiencies in walking.

Just as we need to take into account both the voluntary action and the involuntary reflex reactions of the myofascial system to understand walking, so too must the myofascial system be considered in terms of both individual muscles and interrelated[6] chains of myofascial units. These chains allow a long section of the body—rather than, say, an individual muscle in the leg—to contribute to shock absorption and its control, and this provides longer elastic chains that absorb kinetic energy and then recoil with elastic force,

[6]I use *interrelated* rather than *interconnected*, as not all the proposed lines of continuity are actually continuous and some vary from person to person. However, as shown by van Wingerden et al. 1993, the fascial tissue does not have to be continuous for force transfer across bones; see also chapter 5.

thereby allowing greater energy conservation (see fig. 1.20).

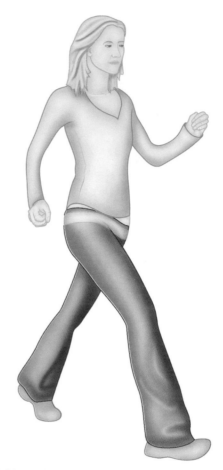

Figure 1.20. At heel strike on the right side, the downward force from the trunk creates a tilt of the pelvis to the left side. This "acceleration" (the sudden tilting to the left) will be perceived and controlled by the hip abductors on the right—the side of heel strike—and the lateral abdominals on the left. Neither the contraction nor the fascial loading will be restricted to just those named muscles but will go further along the lateral aspect of the trunk and thigh.

■ TENSEGRITY

We can now begin to see the interplay between the strength and stability of the skeletal system and the adaptability, buoyancy, and tension abilities of the myofascial system. A tensegrity model of the human body gives us a way of understanding these integrated systems and how they collaborate to distribute tension and organize response (fig. 1.21). "Tensegrity" is at play every time we move; it is inherent within our body as far down as the cellular level, but there are few everyday expressions of it more tangible than the poetic, full-body movement of walking.

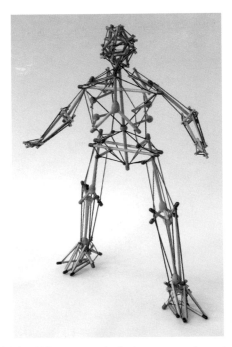

Figure 1.21. *When we see the body represented as a tensegrity system like this, with just the musculoskeletal elements presented (in vague approximation of reality), it is easier to comprehend how the body interacts with its environment to dissipate and produce force.*

The use of relatively solid elements (bone) and elastic elements (myofascia) requires the presence of a certain amount of prestress. It is the contribution of "tension" that gives the structure "integrity" (and it is the combination of these two words that Buckminster Fuller used to coin the term *tensegrity*).

One of the characteristics of tensegrity structures is their ability to distribute stress or changes in tension throughout the whole of the structure. This can be either a positive or a negative thing, depending on the nature of the change. Too much tension will lead to an increase in stiffness and possible breakdown, while a decrease in tension can cause the structure to lose some of its integrity. Balanced tension allows resilience in the system, giving it the ability to disperse, communicate, and store forces across itself and still maintain equilibrium. This is the essence of what therapists aim to achieve

when intervening with a patient's gait: we first need to recognize the imbalance or inability to communicate mechanical force, and then, by appropriate intervention, bring resilience to the patient's system.

While there is some debate over the full application of tensegrity in biological structures, there does seem to be an ever-increasing level of acceptance of the concept. Tensegrity gives us a framework to explain many aspects of human and animal movement. In doing so, we have come full circle, once again using the understanding of architectural structure and geometry to describe human form but with a new and improved vocabulary.

Don Ingber, a researcher at Harvard Medical School, was the first to apply this new geometrical concept to the body, beginning in the 1980s. Ingber showed how cellular structure and mechanics can be explained through tensegrity. Cells have their own inner supports, which allow the transfer of mechanical forces. These forces can communicate cell shape to the nucleus and thereby influence cellular expressions (Ingber 1998).

Steven Levin, a retired orthopedic surgeon, took this a step further and demonstrated that the pelvic and shoulder girdles and the knee joint use similar engineering principles. He argues that tensegrity is the essential building mechanism at the cellular level, the tissue level, and the entire body level. Adding to Ingber's ideas on the laws of self-assembly (the ways in which the cells combine), many consider that tensegrity elements will follow their natural mechanics and attach to one another to grow ever more complex communities, all following the principles of "tensional integrity."

For example, the sacrum is often illustrated as a keystone that gives the pelvis a compressional locking force, using the cumulative weight of the bones from above to hold the pelvis together. Alternatively, a contrary view I was given many years ago presented the sacrum as

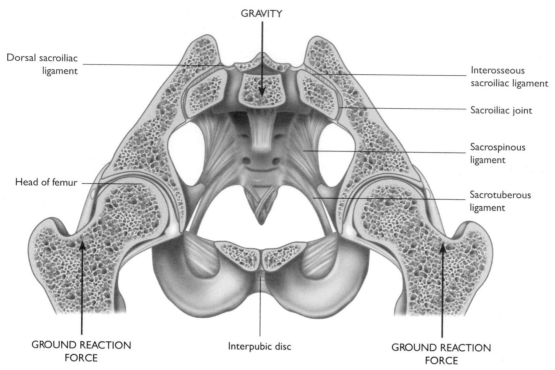

GRAVITY

Dorsal sacroiliac ligament

Interosseous sacroiliac ligament

Sacroiliac joint

Sacrospinous ligament

Head of femur

Sacrotuberous ligament

GROUND REACTION FORCE

Interpubic disc

GROUND REACTION FORCE

Figure 1.22. *When seen in cross section, it is clear that the sacrum is suspended from the ilia, like a hammock between the trees of the ilia; the dorsal sacroiliac ligaments are akin to the ropes of the hammock. Levin argues that the sacrum has to act within the joints to mediate the various forces coming from above and below—gravity and ground reaction force. Furthermore, he argues that the sacrum is supported in the tension created by the "approximation" force (the force that draws two sides together) of the dorsal sacroiliac ligaments, rather than by the compression of the ilia. That is, it is a tensegrity structure (in Vleeming et al. 2007).*

an arrowhead that would split the two sides of the pelvis apart. When the pelvis is examined in cross section (see fig. 1.22), however, the sacrum is clearly shown to be suspended between the ilia. It therefore helps draw the two sides of the pelvis together, using tension from the myofascial guide-wires. In chapter 5, we will see that the "flotation" of the sacrum between the ilia is essential in mediating the many forces that come from the upper and lower bodies. The sacroiliac joints act as a hub for force mediation through the pelvis.

As discussed above, any force applied to a tensegrity structure is dispersed through its entirety, and when we look more closely at distortion, we see two very important phenomena. The first is that tension elements align themselves along the line of pull, helping to increase resistance along that line—effectively making the structure stiffer (and therefore stronger) as more lines are recruited to oppose the stress. This is an

important feature of many biological tissues— they get stiffer under stress, meaning that the stronger the force, the more resistance they have.

A second characteristic of tensegrity structures is that once the strain is removed, the structure returns to its normal resting balance. Tensegrity structures are therefore self-supporting, not requiring the addition of gravity to maintain or hold their form (compared to a tower of blocks, which requires the compression of gravity and loses all integrity when turned at an angle to gravity). Tensegrity structures have an internal resilience that absorbs the energy of external forces and then uses it to return to neutral. The human body applies this dynamic in efficient walking, using the interaction of momentum, gravity, and the resistance from the ground to tension the tissues, and as the body position changes, this tension is released to assist with the return movement, somewhat like a watch-spring mechanism.

■ TRIANGULATION

By standing upright, humans have taken fuller advantage of one of tensegrity's dynamic characteristics. We are less stable by having only two contact points with the ground, and we further exacerbate that instability by balancing on one leg during 80 percent of walking and 100 percent of running (excluding the flight phase of running, when we have no contact with the ground). To manage this acrobatic act, we have changed the way in which the forces pass through the body, allowing much more three-dimensional variation.

In the tensegrity of the upright body, the compression elements (the bones) are supported by the elastic tensioning forces (the myofascia). The vectors of support are arranged in a triangulated pattern following mathematical laws similar to those of crystal formation. As Levin shows (in Vleeming et al. 2007), a triangular truss is much more able to disperse force within itself than a square frame (see fig. 1.23). This is important to keep

in mind, as the body rarely uses movement in just one plane of motion, making it difficult to track events as we go through a movement. Tension is created in each plane: frontal, sagittal, and transverse. I will simplify this in the text by dealing with each in turn, but they are all acting simultaneously.

When tensions in the body are balanced, there is a sense of effortlessness; "compression elements become small islands in a sea of tension" (Buckminster Fuller 1961), and any changes in that equilibrium will be easily absorbed and recoiled back with the natural resilience of the tissue. It is easy for us to imagine the muscular system as the controllers of this tensioning, but the muscles are only one element of the supportive tissues that hold the bones in place. The muscles are essentially the fine-tuners of the system, adding or subtracting tension when needed, via the fascial tissues of the body.

■ FASCIAL MEMBRANES

As mentioned earlier, each and every part of the body is wrapped within the fibrous fascial web of connective tissue, which consists predominantly of collagen, elastin, and ground substance (a gel-like fluid consisting of water along with various sugars and proteins). The fascia holds every single part of our body together and it provides us with protection, both mechanical and chemical—the fascia forms a physical barrier, and the fluid within the fascia contains many lymphocytes. The fibrous elements allow the transfer of force (created either by muscle contractions or by external forces), but they do so with an element of elasticity, which gives us the "spring in our step." This pliability is enhanced through the engagement of longer lines of tissue.

Force is most often considered in terms of straight lines, along muscle fibers and out into tendons and ligaments. This bias is inherent within most anatomy presentations,

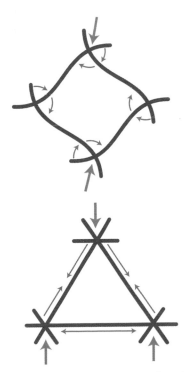

Figure 1.23. A square-based arrangement will tend to buckle under stress, compared to a triangulated structure, which is able to deal with both compression and tension in its structural members.

but it is a misunderstanding, as we need a further appreciation of fascial aponeuroses. Many of the fascial wrapping sheaths in the body are extensions of muscular tissue. These often play an important role in dispersing force by acting as "hydraulic amplifiers" (Gracovetsky 2008; DeRosa and Porterfield, in Vleeming et al. 2007). To understand a "hydraulic amplifier," imagine the example of a balloon. The tension of the outer rubber membrane and the compression of the air inside it create a circumferential "stiffening" dynamic within the structure. If the balloon is not fully inflated, however, there will be little tension created on the outside. The balloon will be less

resilient and will mold itself to the surface it is resting on, rather than being independently buoyant on it. Conversely, if the balloon is overinflated, the elastic will fatigue and lose its ability to adapt to the tension—eventually, it will burst. In the fascia, the body's encasing material, similar events can occur.

This has been studied primarily in the thoracolumbar and thigh areas, where the muscles of the pelvis and the lower back are dealing with high stress loads in various vectors of force and at different anatomical depths (see fig. 1.24). In cross section, we can see the continuity of the posterior

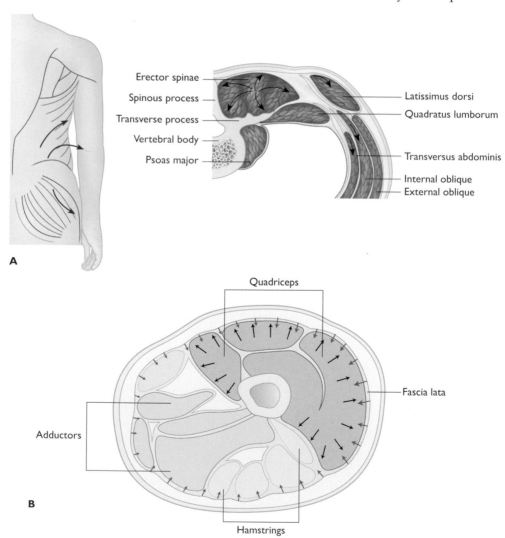

Erector spinae
Spinous process
Transverse process
Vertebral body
Psoas major

Latissimus dorsi
Quadratus lumborum
Transversus abdominis
Internal oblique
External oblique

A

Quadriceps
Fascia lata
Adductors
Hamstrings

B

Figure 1.24. *In walking, the thoracolumbar fascia will be tensioned by the contralateral contraction of the gluteus maximus and latissimus dorsi. This creates tension in the supporting fascia around the lower back muscles, which in turn "pump up" the fascia by pushing out against it when they contract to support the spine (A). This creates a force-dispersal system and is a mechanism used in various parts of the body, including the thigh (B). The enveloping fascia of the thigh, the fascia lata, is tensioned by the appropriately named tensor fasciae latae (TFL) and by the gluteus maximus. Both of those muscles are, in fact, encased within that layer of fascial tissue. This inward force is then met by the outward expansion of the underlying muscles, which will be contracting to support the knee and hip.*

and middle layers of the thoracolumbar fascia wrapping around the muscles—stabilizing, supporting, or moving the lower back.

The contralateral pattern of walking creates tensioning across the diagonal line of the gluteus maximus to the opposite latissimus dorsi muscles via the thoracolumbar fascia (TLF, Willard et al. 2012). The fascial sheet of the TLF and its deeper connections will therefore be tensioned, like the skin of a balloon, and this "shrink wrapping" force will meet the expansion of the muscles within it, creating a taut "balloon" capable of easy force transfer and recoil. It is estimated that this form of hydraulic amplifier can increase the efficiency of muscle contractions by up to 30 percent, though if the fascial sheets are challenged, as in a fasciotomy (the cutting of the fascia to relieve underlying pressure), efficiency can be decreased by 10 to 16 percent (Parker and Briggs 2007).

All of these myofascial layers, while separate in terms of depth and the forces they carry, are connected to one another by a different kind of fluid-rich fascial tissue, known as *areolar* or *loose connective tissue* (fig. 1.25); it provides the lubrication within the system that enables each plane to glide on its neighbor. This tissue,

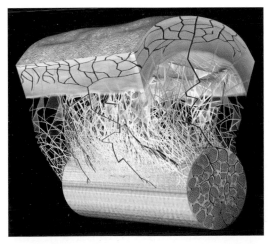

Figure 1.25. *The very fluid areolar tissue contains collagen and elastin fibers, like fascia, but within a much higher concentration of ground substance. This compliant tissue connects fascial layers and facilitates movement by adapting its orientation to the vector of forces involved. (Reproduced with the kind permission of Dr. J. C. Guimberteau and Endovivo Productions.)*

however, is prone to changes in local hydration, creating adhesions which inhibit the relative movement between the different planes.

■ FASCIAL EFFICIENCY

I can remember walking as a child. It was not customary to say you were fatigued. It was customary to complete the goal of the expedition.

—Katharine Hepburn

Appreciating the role of fascia in walking leads us to a new understanding of muscles. The old idea of movement via concentric, eccentric, and occasional isometric contraction is simply not how the body works in many functions. The muscles work as a stiffness-adjusting system. Just as a Pilates instructor changes the springs on a reformer to suit the client or the exercise, so too does the neuromyofascial system adjust the springs to match the forces in the tissue, a constant computational task and one that we still fail to fully understand.

As discussed above, the body needs something to hold it together; it is a bag of bones that, because of their slippery ends, require additional support from the surrounding tissue. The joints—the interfaces between the bones—fold, bend, flex, rotate, or extend in predictable directions. They are therefore able to guide the forces in the body: when the quadriceps contracts, the force is transmitted via the patella to extend the knee. However, when we look at the interaction between the body and the ground, the relationship is reversed: it is the bending of the knee on impact that sends the force to the quadriceps, sparking its contraction.

This reversal of function is important. When we look at movements involving some form of impact with a surface, it is the channeling effect of the joint that creates the movement, not the muscle. The joints are like dry riverbeds that direct the water through the landscape via the path of least resistance. Any movement that creates a normal impact on the body, such as the heel strike in walking, will require the deceleration of momentum (and I will outline the many ways the body does this in the next chapter by tracing the action across the major joints involved in walking).

Using the conventional eccentric/concentric contractions of muscles for each step would require a large amount of resources. The body would have to constantly bind and unbind the actin and myosin filaments of the muscles. We often feel the effects of this muscular type of movement when we go for strolls involving a lot of stopping and starting, such as meandering around a museum or shopping with loved ones on a Saturday afternoon. The constant stopping and starting requires more muscular effort and is therefore much more tiring than going for a long, evenly paced walk, which allows other, more efficient, mechanisms to come into play.

In the repetitive motions of walking, the inner tuning of our springs is unconscious. Apparently even the spinal cord is rarely involved in controlling the movement— it is the local relationship between the mechanoreceptors in the fascial tissue and the surrounding "adjusters" of the muscles that are in charge (see also p. 163, 'Mechanoreceptors – the internal monitors'). By finding the most efficient level of stiffness, the body can maximize the use of elastic recoil and minimize the metabolic costs.

Deformation and Elasticity

Could the young but realize how soon they will become mere walking bundles of habits, they would give more heed to their conduct while in the plastic state.

—William James

As we saw in the Fukunaga experiments reported earlier (see fig. 1.14), the force-guiding effect of the joints will lead to *deformation* of the myofascia in repetitive motions such as walking. *Deformation* is defined as any compression, shear, or tension. We will concentrate on the production of tension that stresses the tissues and thereby lengthens them. The amount tissue lengthens depends on a number of factors, including age, hydration, and nutrition, but it also depends on the quality of that tissue, as not all myofascia is the same. Some myofascia will have more connective tissue, and this will affect its elasticity (its ability to lengthen and return to its original position). For example, there is an obvious difference in the architecture of the gastrocnemius, the sartorius, and the semimembranosus (see fig. 1.26). The passive force curve (which measures the elasticity of the connective tissue in each muscle) illustrates the greater stiffness of the gastrocnemius and shows how its resistance to stretch begins sooner than in the sartorius or semimembranosus. This means that the connective tissue of the gastrocnemius is stretched earlier in its movement, and it requires more energy to be lengthened, an important feature for economy of gait.

By elongating the connective tissue of the gastrocnemius, for example, we are creating a store of energy. Most organic materials have some form or amount of elastic ability; they are able to strain (deform) and then return to their original length. The obvious example is a rubber band, which requires stress to stretch but will then recoil to its original state by itself. If you pull a rubber band, you feel the energy required to stretch it, and if it snaps back against your fingers, you will certainly experience the energy available in the return. In the case of the body's movement in walking, the elastic tissue is stretched ("loaded") through its interaction with the natural pressures of gravity, ground reaction force, and momentum.

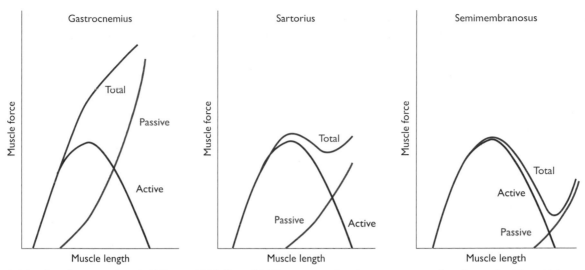

Figure 1.26. *Based on work done by Wilkie in 1968, Komi (2011) points out that the gastrocnemius has shorter fascicles, which means that it will be less able to stretch than the longer-fibered thigh muscles of the sartorius and semimembranosus. This will send the force of that stretch into the gastrocnemius's connective tissue at a shorter range of motion (the gastrocnemius has more connective tissue for this reason). Areas of the body with higher mechanical stress will use a number of strategies to deal with the extra loading. One of those is a greater amount of connective tissue, which protects the area and allows the force to be absorbed and returned as energy. We will also see later that pennate muscles, in which the muscle fibers attach to the tendon at an oblique angle, add efficiency to this system.*

The amount of energy returned in the recoil does not always match the energy that was initially created (some energy is lost in the system), but in terms of economy, connective tissue is quite efficient: up to 93 percent of energy is returned to the system. This means that a lot of the energy being used in walking is almost "free"—it does not require the active contraction of the muscles and the use of oxygen. Some measurements have indicated that about 17 percent of the force required in running originates from the recoil of the arches of the feet, while 16 percent in walking comes from the Achilles tendon (Blazevich 2011).

The loss of energy from the system, or the hysteresis effect (see figs. 1.27 and 1.11), is due to the *viscosity* of the tissue, which is its resistance to deformation. Viscosity varies considerably, depending on the chemical nature and makeup of the tissues involved, all of which can also create a slight delay in tissue recoil.

Viscoelasticity

The viscosity within the connective tissue is a double-edged sword: not only does it rob us of

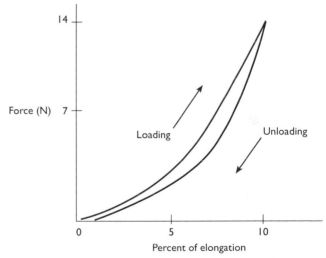

Figure 1.27. *The graph illustrates the nonlinear nature of the amount of force required to stretch connective tissue (i.e., more force is required for the second centimeter of stretch than for the first centimeter). The blue line maps the tissue's elastic return to resting length. In a truly efficient system, the two lines would match (i.e., the same force would return to the system). The gap between the two lines illustrates the lost energy due to hysteresis, an inherent property of the tissue.*

some of the available recoil energy, but it also absorbs a portion of the body's momentum, particularly in its struggle against gravity, and by doing so, it removes some of the workload from the muscles. Connective tissue is often referred to as *viscoelastic* because of this combination of properties.

The fluid element within fascia, the ground substance, is made up of proteins and sugars (glycosaminoglycans) and behaves in a nonlinear fashion. Sometimes referred to as a *non-Newtonian fluid* (so called because it does not react to forces in a linear, "Newton-approach" fashion), the ground substance can become "stickier" and, when force is applied at speed, can provide more stiffness for the system.

You may have felt this reaction when comparing a Hatha yoga–type slow stretch to a plyometric exercise. The sharper, faster movements of the plyometrics create a strong and often linear response in the tissue compared to when movement is entered into slowly, which has a more dispersed effect. The viscosity can be affected by a number of factors, including heat (compare a Bikram yoga class to stretching at the North Pole) and the

hydration of the tissue (the ground substance is extremely hydrophilic and needs to bind to water molecules to maintain fluidity). This mechanism comes into play during walking: when a joint is encouraged to move in the deceleration phase—after heel strike, when the system is working to absorb the force of gravity and the ground reaction force—the viscous ground substance will stiffen the tissue and thereby allow the fascial fibers to load more, taking further advantage of the elastic recoil.

Stretch Reflex

The elastic stretching of the tissue also stimulates many of the body's mechanoreceptors, the proprioceptors for the body. The muscle spindle in particular, sensing the stretch within the myofascia, will set off the stretch reflex arc (see fig. 1.28).

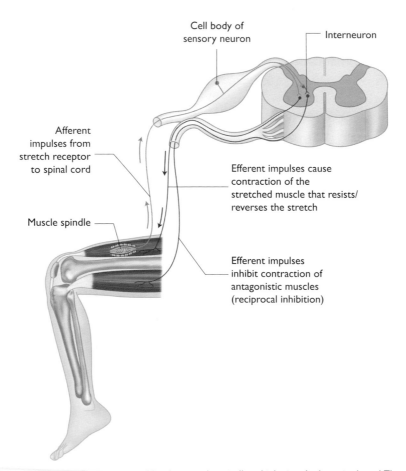

Cell body of sensory neuron

Interneuron

Afferent impulses from stretch receptor to spinal cord

Efferent impulses cause contraction of the stretched muscle that resists/reverses the stretch

Muscle spindle

Efferent impulses inhibit contraction of antagonistic muscles (reciprocal inhibition)

Figure 1.28. The lengthening of the myofascia is sensed by the muscle spindle, which signals the spinal cord. The spinal cord responds with an efferent (motor) nerve signal for the muscle to contract.

The reflex arc creates the contraction of the muscle, which is predominantly isometric. Further deceleration of the body's movement then loads the connective tissue, which eventually reaches a point at which the force required to lengthen it further has been absorbed by the increasing stiffness of the elastic fiber. Once it reaches the stage at which the force stretching the fiber equals the tension within it, it begins to recoil, just like a weight bouncing on the end of a spring. The amount of energy lost by the system can depend on the period of time spent at the end of range. This amortization, or transition phase, will affect the amount of recoil.

Exercise 1.2. **Amortization Exercise**

These three jumping exercises illustrate the variations and differences in the loading of elastic tissue. Just notice what feels right for your own body, as well as noticing what height you attain with each jump.

A. First try jumping without first bringing your head closer to the floor (i.e., do not bend your knees before the jump). This is difficult, as you will only be able to rely on the power of your ankle plantar flexors. Notice how high you are able to get from the floor with just those muscles.

B. Now bend your knees and stay for a moment in the flexed position before jumping. In this jump, you will be able to take advantage of the power of the hip and knee extensors as well as your lower leg muscles.

C. Finally, bend your knees as in B, but jump in a flowing movement, coming down further, into a squat, and then almost immediately pushing up (as you probably wanted to in jump B). You will feel the benefit of the additional elastic recoil.

The jump in B added the strong thigh muscles but did not include the additional energy of elastic loading, because too much time was spent in the transition phase. This is also one of the effects of "museum walking": the stop-and-start nature of it takes away the free energy of the elastic tissue. Rhythm is therefore important, and this can be felt in actions such as jumping and hopping: when done too slowly or too quickly the effort becomes muscular, but somewhere in the middle, the movement will take advantage of elastic recoil and will feel "just right."

That is not to say no muscle energy will be involved, just that the ratio will favor elasticity. And, of course, it will also depend on the activity being done and the person's tissue type, as well as which myofascial areas are being tensioned.

Rhythm will influence the amount of energy we can garner from the fascial tissues (as seen in exercise 1.2). This can vary significantly from person to person and will depend on a variety of factors, including tissue type (loosely or tightly ligamented, for example), hydration, age, and the general condition of the tissue. A number of experiments have looked at the reasons why we use different types of movement at different speeds. A walk uses a different movement strategy from that for a run, and they both differ from that for a sprint. Studies of energy usage have found that whenever the movement style is changed to match the speed of movement, there is a recovery of efficiency—i.e., less energy is used.

Running at a low speed is less efficient than walking, because of the way the tissues are being loaded. The lower efficiency is probably due to the increased time in the transition phase, because the longer stride in running increases downward momentum, forcing the muscles to work to recover. Walking with less upward/downward movement compared to running is only efficient at speeds of up to 7.25 to 7.4 kilometers per hour, at which point we tend to switch to running (McArdle 2010). The increased speed of the run will utilize

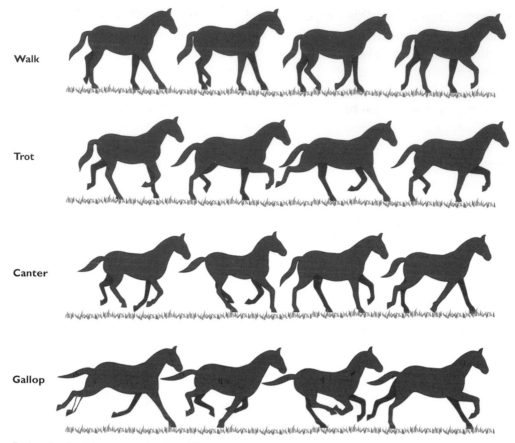

Figure 1.29. *Each style of gait is associated with a different pattern of body use. Changing the length of the stride is one of many strategies to maximize efficiency at each "gear change."*

the up/down loading into the tissue, and the amount of time in the transition phase will be reduced. This has been studied in horses, as they change their style of gait from walk to trot to canter and, finally, to gallop (fig. 1.29). The gradual increase in the horse's speed inevitably leads to an increase in muscle work, but with each gait change, there is a recovery of relative efficiency by taking advantage of more elastic energy being returned from the fascial tissue (Biewener 1998).

Different movement strategies are used at various speeds to maintain elastic efficiency, but so too must we adapt to other changes in the forces of gravity and ground reaction. Some studies have shown that certain African women are able to carry up to 20 percent of their own body weight on their heads and still maintain the same efficiency in walking (Maloiy et al. 1986; McArdle 2010). The analysis of the reasons for this is not fully complete, but

it seems that the women are able to transform the increased downward momentum caused by the extra weight into elastic energy rather than recruiting additional muscle effort. We will see how the displacement of body weight can assist elastic loading and recoil throughout the book. Rhythm, momentum and tissue type can then combine to minimize the hysteresis area seen in fig. 1.1 for maximum efficiency during movement.

■ THE STRETCH-SHORTENING CYCLE AND WALKING

The stretch-shortening cycle is the basis for many normal human activities and utilizes all of the above mechanisms: stretch reflex, elastic recoil, and viscoelasticity. It requires a preparatory movement (or a countermovement) to stimulate the muscle spindles to isometrically contract the muscle, which forces the stretch of the elastic tissues. In walking, this happens through the natural folding of the joints, but in other actions, such as throwing, it is achieved through a countermovement, using the opposite action to load the tissues; for certain movements, that will often be faster than muscle contraction alone.

Muscle integrity is important, as the muscle must be strong enough to decelerate movement to ensure that the fascial tissue is stretched by the momentum. Muscle-tendon units do more for the body than simply lengthen and shorten: "they can act as rigid struts to transfer mechanical energy, as a motor to produce mechanical energy, as a damper to dissipate mechanical energy or as a spring to store and return elastic energy" (Sawicki et al. 2009).

All of the roles of the muscle-tendon units have to be coordinated. Any loss of elasticity in one area will lead to increased muscle work in another. For example, imagine losing the ability to plantar flex at toe-off, a predominantly elastic mechanism. Some other part of the leg, most likely a muscle, would have to compensate for that loss of kinetic energy, and that concentric muscle contraction would have metabolic costs.

■ SUMMARY

1. To support the energy demands of the brain, the human body tries to minimize the number of calories consumed by muscle work.
2. The development of upright gait freed our hands for other tasks, many of which had calorie-saving or calorie-consuming benefits.
3. Upright stance brought our skeleton into closer alignment with gravity, reducing joint flexions and improving our mechanical advantage.
4. The stretch-shortening cycle is our preferred method of motivation in normal everyday movement. The alternative—the constant elongation and shortening of muscles—requires repeated engagement and release of the actin and myosin elements, which increases the energy demands for movement. The stretch-shortening cycle reduces overall metabolic cost by taking advantage of three mechanisms: the tissue's viscoelasticity, to begin the deceleration; the stretch reflex, to isometrically contract the muscle tissue; and the elastic lengthening and recoil of the fascial tissues.
5. The body has a natural variation in the design of myofascial structures within it. Appropriate movement strategies will take advantage of each tissue's natural design to increase the efficiency of the movement.
6. Fascial tissues help disperse force and maximize elastic loading but require enough range of motion at various joints to facilitate force transfer.
7. By "triangulating"—using a combination of these lines of force—the body also gains more effective control over movement than it would do if it relied on just one. Incorporating forces from slightly different angles allows finer control in response to deviating influences.
8. When any part of the body impacts with a surface (most often the foot with the ground), the orientation of the joints serves to send the force of the impact into soft tissues along predictable channels. These channels have presumably adapted over time and function to spread the stress into tissues with the appropriate muscle fiber and fascial architecture.
9. The predictable order and direction of the folding in the joints then creates the proper conditions to tension the myofascial tissue for greatest economy in their return movement.

2

THE MECHANICAL CHAIN

If you seek creative ideas go walking. Angels whisper to a man when he goes for a walk.

—Raymond I. Myers

■ INTRODUCTION

There are lots of reasons why we move the way that we do. Chapter one introduced us to many of the evolutionary and economical advantages of myofascial strategies, and we will continue to build that vision by breaking down the movements and complexities of each phase of gait. Some examples from comparative anatomy will be used to enhance our understanding of the relationship between form and function. We will look at how the interweaving of the forces, the joint abilities and alignments, and the soft tissues creates a symbiotic flow through the walking body.

We will introduce the functions of walking then explore the phases of gait and their implications. Each phase of the gait cycle creates new demands on the body, but our system is adapted to take advantage of the stresses—provided our tissues are able to cooperate. The foot is a main area of stress

during gait, as it has to provide mobility and stability at different stages. We will examine the mechanics used by the foot to both distribute and control force.

A description of movement is difficult and can be confusing, and so in this chapter we define real and relative movement, also known as *osteokinematics* and *arthrokinematics*, to help clarify what is really happening and when. Familiarity with these terms and concepts will not only assist the reader with progressing through the book but also provide clarity when analyzing any complex movement.

■ FUNCTIONS OF WALKING

Perry (2010) lists four functions of walking: propulsion, energy conservation, stance stability, and shock absorption. Each of them helps to clarify the role of the soft tissues in walking.

Propulsion

Much of human movement is goal oriented: we think of a desired outcome, and our body takes us toward it (remember that walking is often a method of getting our head or hands to where we want them). We do not have the space and energy in our conscious minds to sequentially send each and every signal to the relevant musculature. Instead, as demonstrated in the previous chapter, humans allow the somatic nervous system to take over the jobs of initiation and direct propulsion.

To understand propulsion, we have to know about both the voluntary and the reflex actions and abilities of the myofascial system. As explained in chapter 1, the natural folding patterns of the joints sends the force of the movement into the channels of the soft tissue, causing a reaction in the local proprioceptive reflexes embedded and hardwired in the fascial tissue. These reflexes give localized and rapid control in response to the forces experienced in the local communication system, reducing the need for signals to be sent all the way up to the spinal cord or—causing even more delay—to the brain and back.

Energy Conservation

It is tempting to view propulsion as a consistent and alternating series of concentric/eccentric contractions; however, once propulsion has started, momentum provides much of the energy required in a flat repetitive gait, and it is momentum that provides our locomotor economy. The primary mechanism for the recycling of energy was explored in the previous chapter, but it is worth repeating here that the elastic tissues load energy they receive from external sources (which can include muscle contraction), and that the main provider of energy will be momentum. Compared to quadrupeds, more of our tissues are involved during gait as a result of the stacked, upright skeleton's ability to vault over the foot because of the stability provided by the skeletal alignment.

Stance Stability

For us to walk on two legs, we have to be able to stand on one leg and vault over the

planted foot. Our success in this acrobatic act required us to align our center of gravity above our point of contact with the ground; to achieve this, human anatomy has evolved in many ways. Following on from the alignment modifications of the ilia, another major change is the carrying angle between the hip joint and the knee: the human leg angles inward to allow the feet to align more closely with the midline and the body's center of gravity. In nonhuman primates, there is very little approximation of the knees and feet, meaning that their lower legs lie fairly lateral to the line of gravity, making it much more likely that they would fall if they were to stand on one leg (see fig. 2.1).

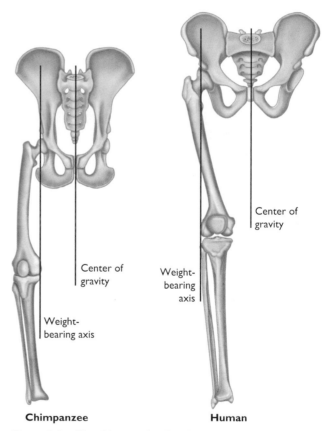

Chimpanzee   **Human**

Figure 2.1. The oblique angle of the human leg allows the support of the body's center of gravity to be brought closer in alignment to its supporting leg. The vertical angle of the nonhuman primate leg maintains that line of force medial to the support when standing on one leg.

Stability is enhanced in humans by the posterior aspect of the human ilium facing more laterally than that of nonhuman primates (see fig. 2.2). The fascicular direction of the gluteal muscles is altered and they can therefore act in abducting as well as extending the hip. Abduction—or should we call it *prevention of adduction*?—is vital to the ability to stand on one leg. Much of this angle of support is missing from the nonhuman primate pelvis,

which faces posteriorly, making their gluteal muscles primarily extensors—excellent for pushing forward but not great for creating stability in single-leg stance.

When walking, humans move their feet even closer to the midline. The average separation of the feet is 8 centimeters for men and 7 centimeters for women, again helping to bring the line of support below the center of gravity.

Shock Absorption

The natural rise and fall of human gait creates a force of impact following heel strike that needs to be dissipated before reaching the top of the body in order to keep the head relatively steady. The heel strike of a normal gait pattern produces both upward and backward forces that must be controlled. The absorption, dissipation, and recycling of impact forces is an underpinning element of our exploration and an area in which the joints and their alignment with the soft tissue excel.

On impact, the joints will fold naturally, according to the interaction between the ground reaction force, the momentum of the movement, and the location of the body's center of gravity. This natural folding of the joints channels the mechanical information about the impact into the "streams" of the soft tissue to be sensed by the mechanoreceptors encased within the fascia. If the mechanical communication is working, the appropriate muscular forces are activated to prevent collapse.

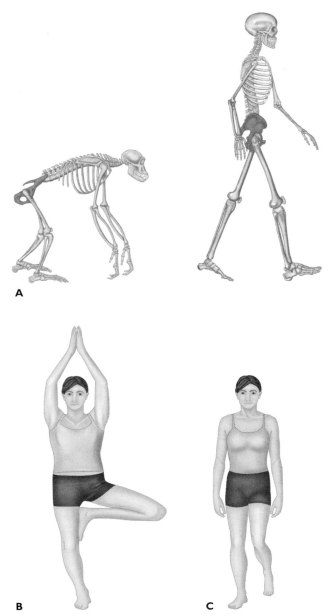

Figure 2.2. *A, We can see the alteration in angle, which took place at some point during evolution, that allowed the hip extensors of the nonhuman primate to face more laterally, thereby creating the ability to stand on one leg, an essential part of bipedal gait. B, To achieve and maintain this pose for any length of time, we can see how the carrying angle described above (the medial placement of the knee and therefore the foot) and the line of force of contraction from the laterally facing abductors help to keep the body's center of gravity from falling to the left. C, Here we see the necessity for lateral stability, as one leg is in contact with the ground while the other swings through into flexion.*

When external forces act across joints, the natural tendency of the joint determines the action of the soft tissue—in other words, the action of the soft tissue is a reaction to the joint's movement. For example, you may have been taught to bend your knees when landing after a jump, but in reality, that is all the knee joints can do; their only other choice

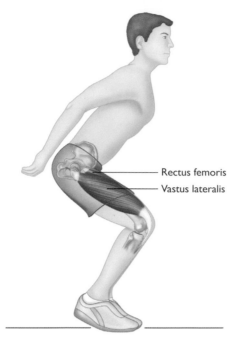

Figure 2.3. *The knees—and many other joints—can allow the myofascial tissue to absorb much of the force of landing from a jump by collapsing along their predetermined vectors. This channels the mechanical force into soft tissue, which can eccentrically lengthen to decelerate the body.*

the downward force, decelerating the body (see fig. 2.3).

As we will see in the biomechanical chain, a number of joints will act to absorb the various forces in the three dimensions, not only maintaining equilibrium, but also assisting with the efficiency of movement. The joints determine the vectors of force coming into the body; those forces are controlled by the neuromyofascial web, and—provided there is the correct stiffness in the surrounding soft tissue—the stresses will be absorbed. However, if there is too much mobility or not enough inherent strength in the musculature, there will be a relative collapse of the joint, potentially causing hypermobility of the joint and creating the need for muscles elsewhere to compensate for the loss in elastic energy.

is to stay straight. The bending of the knee sends the force into the strong quadriceps group, which can act eccentrically to absorb

▪ GAIT CYCLE

One of the difficulties of analyzing gait has always been the continuous three-dimensional changes that occur during the gait cycle.

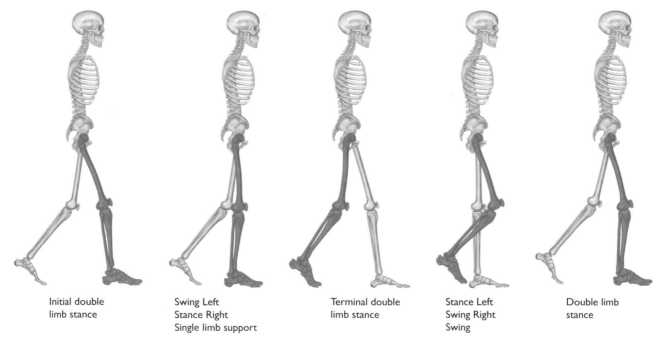

| Initial double limb stance | Swing Left Stance Right Single limb support | Terminal double limb stance | Stance Left Swing Right Swing | Double limb stance |

Figure 2.4. *The divisions of gait. (After Perry and Burnfield 2010.)*

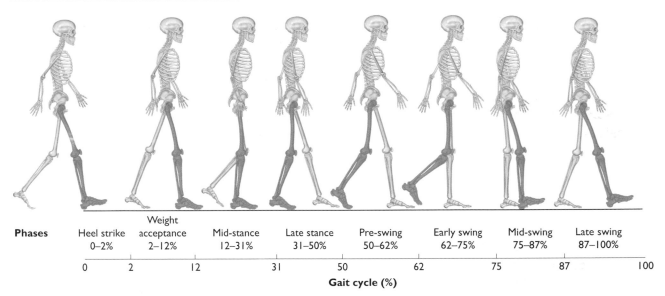

Phases	Heel strike 0–2%	Weight acceptance 2–12%	Mid-stance 12–31%	Late stance 31–50%	Pre-swing 50–62%	Early swing 62–75%	Mid-swing 75–87%	Late swing 87–100%

Gait cycle (%)

Figure 2.5. *Divisions of the gait cycle.*

The eight basic phases[1] we will refer to in this text are: heel strike (0–2%); weight acceptance (2–12%); mid-stance (12–31%); late stance (31–50%); pre-swing (50–62%[2]); early swing (62–75%); mid-swing (75–87%); and late swing (87–100%); after which we return to heel strike. We will use this terminology to describe a full stride, which actually comprises two steps—we start with a right-side heel strike, step forward to a left-side heel strike, and then come back to a heel strike on the right again. A familiarity with the terminology of the periods and phases (figs. 2.4 & 2.5) will serve you well, but it is not essential that you remember them now. As you work through the book and understand what is happening at each phase, the terms will become clear.

One full stride (the gait cycle) consists of a *stance period*, when the foot is on the ground, and a *swing period*, when it passes through the air. The stance period requires weight acceptance and single-limb support to occur during the first four phases, and the swing period occurs from toe-off to heel strike (figs. 2.4 & 2.5).

[1] These phases and their timings are based on Perry and Burnfield (2010); other references in the literature may vary in their application of the timings, but the slight variation is not significant enough to concern us here.

[2] Toe-off will occur at 62%.

■ THE SKELETAL CHAIN

The Role of the Foot

The human foot is a masterpiece of engineering and a work of art.

—Leonardo da Vinci

The spotlight brought to the foot in response to the barefoot running craze has given us a new appreciation of the beautiful and complex engineering at the bottom of our legs. The foot has to be able to handle the forces following heel strike: it must bear our weight, and then create a stable platform from which to launch forward again. To deal with these forces, the foot rolls over a series of rounded bone and joint surfaces from heel to toe (see "Foot Rockers, Force Closure, a Catapult" below) as we vault over the top of it with our various twists and turns. During the transition from heel strike to toe-off, the foot first acts as a stable base then quickly opens and unlocks to absorb and distribute shock; it finally re-establishes its integrity again in preparation for toe-off. The foot's multitasking has given us our long and efficient stride by virtue of its ability to heel strike, weight accept, and toe-off—all through being able to supinate, pronate, and then re-supinate.

As the foot passes from supination (stable) to pronation (open, and adaptable) and back to the stability of supination, it recruits both intrinsic and extrinsic mechanisms to support each transition. By first exploring the intrinsic mechanics of the foot, we will be better placed to understand the importance of the rest of the body during the phases of gait; just like the recurrent supination-pronation-supination cycle of the foot, I recommend cycling back and forth between this section and subsequent chapters to review the interconnections.

The only way to understand a land is to walk it. The only way to drink in its real meaning is to keep it firmly beneath one's feet ... Only the walker can form the wider view.

—Sinclair McKay, *Ramble on: The Story of Our Love for Walking Britain*

Walking with the calcaneus, metatarsals, and toes on the ground (*plantigrady*; see fig 2.6) is not unique to humans; many other animals, such as kangaroos and bears, also use the whole foot in contact with the ground. What is unique to us, however, is the ability to take a long stride on a straight leg. This long stride has required modifications to various bones and joints, and we will explore many of these as we progress through the book. We have already seen one important feature in the lateral orientation of the ilia (see figs. 2.2 and 2.7), but we will explore the foot first.

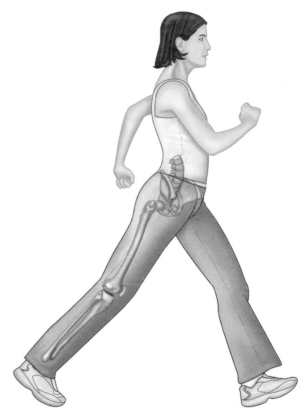

Figure 2.7. *The long stride requires toe extension on the back foot, straight knees on both legs, hip and lumbar extension, and the ability to heel strike with the front foot. To accomplish this, each joint range has required adaptations over time.*

The ability to toe extend is an underpinning criterium for efficient upright gait and is often used to discern locomotor patterns of extinct hominin species. Arboreal primates need to be able to grip rounded surfaces with their digits, a preference demonstrated by the natural "flexion" within the bones of the foot

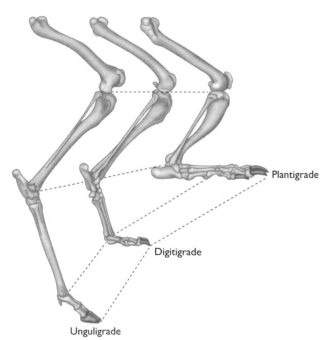

Plantigrade

Digitigrade

Unguligrade

Figure 2.6. *Most other mammals walk on some aspect of their forefoot, either hoofs (unguligrade) or toes (digitigrade). Having the heel connect with the ground allows fewer joints to absorb the forces at impact.*

(see fig. 2.8). *Homo sapiens* possesses straighter metatarsals, which has important implications for our functional range in our upright gait. That importance lies in the relative starting position: it is not the overall range of motion that is important, but rather the starting angle. The distal surface of the metatarsals of the chimpanzee points downward, while that of the human points straight ahead. When the chimpanzee foot is resting on the ground, the metatarsophalangeal (MTP) joint will already be in relative extension and therefore unable to go much further into extension. In contrast, the human MTP joint will rest on the ground in neutral and thereby facilitate the step forward by allowing more movement into extension.

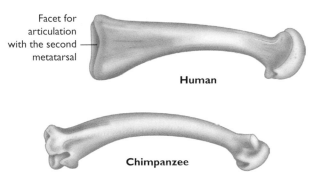

Facet for
articulation
with the second —
metatarsal

Human

Chimpanzee

Figure 2.8.   *Lateral views of the first metatarsal of* Homo sapiens *and* Pan troglodytes. *(Adapted from Aiello and Dean 2002.)*

Human toe extension is also aligned differently from that of other primates (see fig. 2.9). As humans rarely require a grasping big toe, the first ray (medial cuneiform, metatarsal, phalanges, and sesamoids) has adducted and aligned the first and second MTP joints with the sagittal plane. By extending onto the heads of both first and second metatarsals during the toe-off phase, the foot has a relatively stable two-point contact with the ground and, importantly, the movement is aligned with the front of the hip joint.

One can feel the importance of the predominantly sagittal alignment of the MTP joints by stepping forward into a lunge with the feet parallel, and then repeating the lunge with the back foot turned outward. On stepping straight ahead, the stretch experienced at the hip tends to be at the front; when stepping forward with the laterally rotated foot, however, the stretch is felt more toward the inside of the hip, closer to the adductors. This simple exercise demonstrates the importance of MTP joint alignment for the tissue around the hip joint when stepping forward, and illustrates only one of a number of independent joint relationships that will be encountered throughout this text.

Appropriate joint alignment and range of motion are essential in allowing the transfer of momentum to the correct tissues further along the chain. As experienced in the above exercise, incorrect orientation of the foot affects the reaction of the hip, and there must be adequate range of motion at the ankle and toes to allow simultaneous toe extension and hip extension. Toe alignment is less important for the other primates, because they are unable to extend their toes and hips at the same time in the sagittal plane. For humans, on the other hand, the coupling of toe and hip extension in the same plane creates an important efficiency

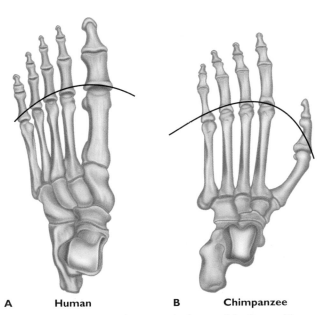

A   **Human**   **B**   **Chimpanzee**

Figure 2.9.   *Numerous changes in the bones of the foot and leg have created a more consistent sagittal alignment in the bones of the human foot (A) compared to other primates (chimpanzee shown for comparison, B). Note the more arced alignment of the chimp's metatarsophalangeal joints. (Adapted from Aiello and Dean 2002.)*

mechanism that allows the hip flexors, plantar flexors, and toe flexors to engage simultaneously and maintain joint integrity during movement.

Alignment of the toe joints, coupled with our upright stance, is a major contributor to our locomotor efficiency. As we progress through the rest of the chapters in this book, we will see that the combined para-sagittal progression over the foot allows momentum to stiffen and strain the numerous tissues crossing the hip and abdomen as we take a long step. The long step requires toe extension on the back foot and the ability to heel strike on the forward foot with a relatively straight leg (fig. 2.7). Striking with a straight leg, however, requires some form of shock absorption to prevent brain-rattling vibrations from occurring.

As discussed in the previous chapter, lighter animals use a series of bends in their joints during locomotion, but, as we saw, that is a metabolically expensive strategy. Our straight-leg alternative allows skeletal alignment to reduce the work during gait, as there are a few areas where our anatomy has relative bends and offsets that allow shock absorption; however, a high effective mechanical advantage (EMA) is maintained by keeping the offsets to a minimum.

One obvious area of shock absorption is the arched arrangement of the human foot (see fig. 2.10). The raised plantar surface is filled with many tough tissues and allows the foot to open and spread into pronation following heel strike. Pronation serves many functions: it unlocks the joints, gives the foot some adaptability to mold to the walking surface, and loads energy into the plantar tissues.

Toe alignment and the arched formation of the foot are structurally related. When compared to other primates, human tibias show a greater degree of lateral torsion, which has affected the angle of the first ray and the axis of the

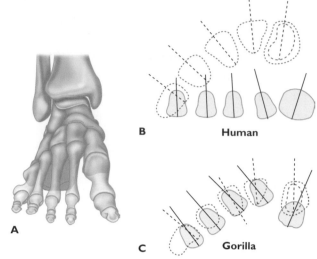

Figure 2.10. *The placement of the metatarsal bases and heads of a human (A and B) and a gorilla (C). The human metatarsal heads are lower and can rest on the ground, with their proximal portions raised as part of the dome arrangement of the foot. The metatarsals of the gorilla remain in the same plane, indicating a flat foot. (Images B and C from Aiello and Dean 2002.)*

subtalar joint (see fig. 2.11). Tibial torsion plays an important role in positioning the foot: when the tibia turns laterally, the corresponding foot supinates; conversely, when the tibia medially rotates, the foot pronates. This transverse plane relationship is coupled via the tibiotalar joint (see fig. 2.10A). The tibiotalar joint is aligned so as to facilitate plantar flexion and dorsiflexion; however, because of the overlapping of the talus by the medial and lateral malleoli, the joint has only a few degrees of rotation available to it. As a result of this reduced transverse plane freedom at the tibiotalar joint, the transverse movement of one bone (talus, fibula, or tibia) transfers to the other in a coupling action.

The coupling of movement across joints is another underpinning element in our locomotor pattern and, once again, is something we will build during the rest of the book. In the case of the tibiotalar joint, we will see the foot's adaptation to the ground causes a predictable sequence of reactions upward through the lower limb; the foot then responds to rotation of the lower limb in the opposite direction during the late stance phase.

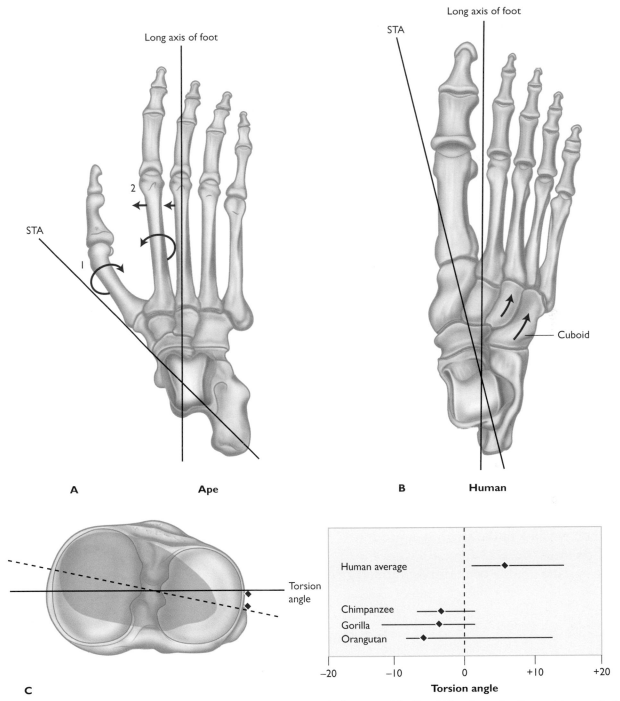

Figure 2.11. A, The axis of the subtalar joint has been brought closer to the long axis of the foot. B, The change in alignment has resulted from an increase in length of the cuboid and lateral cuneiform and lateral torsion of the tibia. C, The change in subtalar angle has been assisted by the greater lateral torsion of the tibia in humans compared to that in other primates.

The normal descriptive terminology for the arched arrangement of the foot does not do it justice. The intricate and interrelated form of the lower limb (indeed of the rest of the body, but we will limit ourselves to the foot and leg for the moment) requires us to see beyond the idea of medial, lateral, and transverse arches, and consider the foot as one functional half-dome. The concept of a half-dome was first introduced by McKenzie in 1955 and recently revived in an article by McKeon et al. (2015; see fig. 2.12). Considering the foot as a functional unit makes sense, as it is impossible to isolate any one aspect of the foot during movement—the whole foot responds during any movement.

Admittedly, some aspects of this functional unit may respond more or less than others, but the reality is that the whole limb is constantly reacting to its force environment, as illustrated by the uninterrupted trabecular pattern passing from one bone to another in fig. 2.12B.

In his prescient and wide-ranging text *On Growth and Form*, D'Arcy Wentworth Thompson explored the significance of variation in trabecular patterns between species. He describes the human ankle arrangement as "two compression members sloping apart from one another; and these have to be bound together by a 'tie' or tension-member, corresponding to the third, horizontal member of the truss" (Thompson 1940, page 980). The use of tension and compression members to describe anatomy in the second edition of the book, published in 1942, predates Kenneth Snelson's first structures by six years and gives a perfect image of the body's use of triangulation for stability and mobility.

The half-dome arrangement has provided the human foot with the ability to twist and untwist in response to the forces acting through it. When we look at the rhythm of ground reaction force (fig. 2.13A and B), we see a characteristic double peak during human gait which is quite different from that shown for the other primates. The two peaks correspond to heel strike and toe-off and can also be seen on the plantar pressure reading (fig. 2.13C). The foot needs to be stable during these peaks but also has to dissipate some of the forces during the stages in between.

The offset between the talus and the calcaneus also leads to an offset between the forces of mass and momentum coming down the limb to the talus and the ground reaction force (as mentioned in chapter 1) coming up from the calcaneus as it strikes the ground. The offset forces cause the calcaneus to evert (or, medially tilt) following heel strike. Calcaneal eversion tilts the sustentaculum talus, and the talus bone then glides down the sustentaculum talus and medially rotates (fig. 2.14). The medial rotation of the talus is key to the reaction of the foot distally and to the lower limb proximally, because of the coupling effect of the tibiotalar joint.

The double peak of the ground reaction force shown in fig. 2.13A illustrates the foot's ability to transition from a rigid lever (peak) to a mobile adaptor (trough) and return to a rigid lever (peak) again. Other primates have "chosen" flexibility and mobility for their feet (an advantage in arboreal behavior), and their

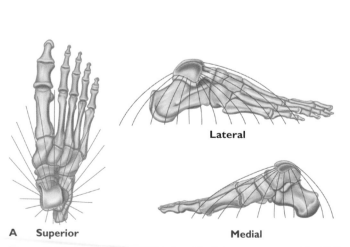

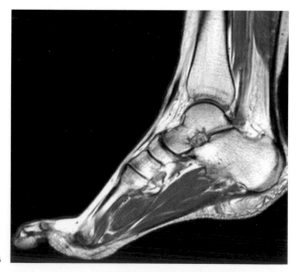

A   **Superior**   **Lateral**   **Medial**   B

Figure 2.12.   *A, The foot as a functional half-dome, as proposed by McKenzie, 1955 in McKeon et al. 2014. B, An X-ray showing the continuity of the trabecular pattern.*

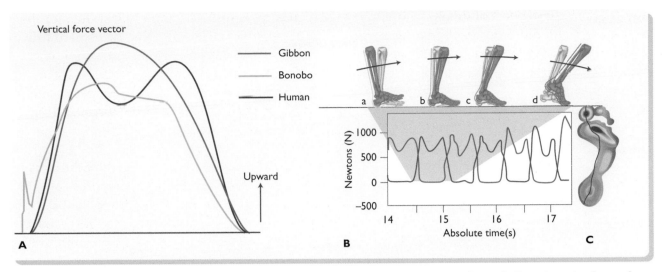

Figure 2.13.   *A, Comparison of ground reaction forces of a human, gibbon, and bonobo during upright gait. B, Ground reaction forces of the left (green) and the right (purple) foot during normal gait, showing the alternating rhythm with characteristic double peaks following heel strike and before toe-off. The shaded section relates to one stance phase, from heel strike to toe-off. C, Plantar pressure readings. (Adapted from Crompton et al. 2008.)*

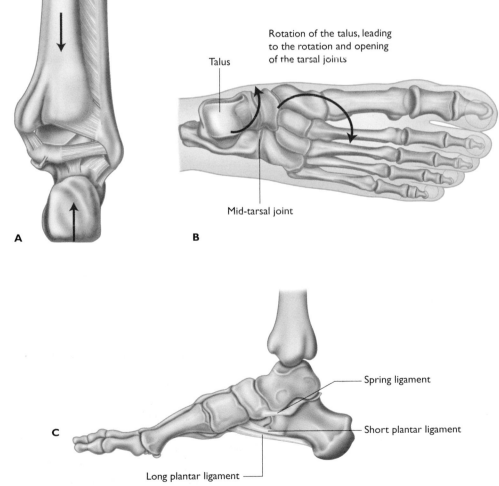

Figure 2.14.   *The offset between the calcaneus and the talus (A) causes the calcaneus to evert following heel strike. The rotation of the talus unlocks the midtarsal joints of the foot (B) and allows the plantar tissues (particularly the ligaments shown in C) to absorb much of the shock.*

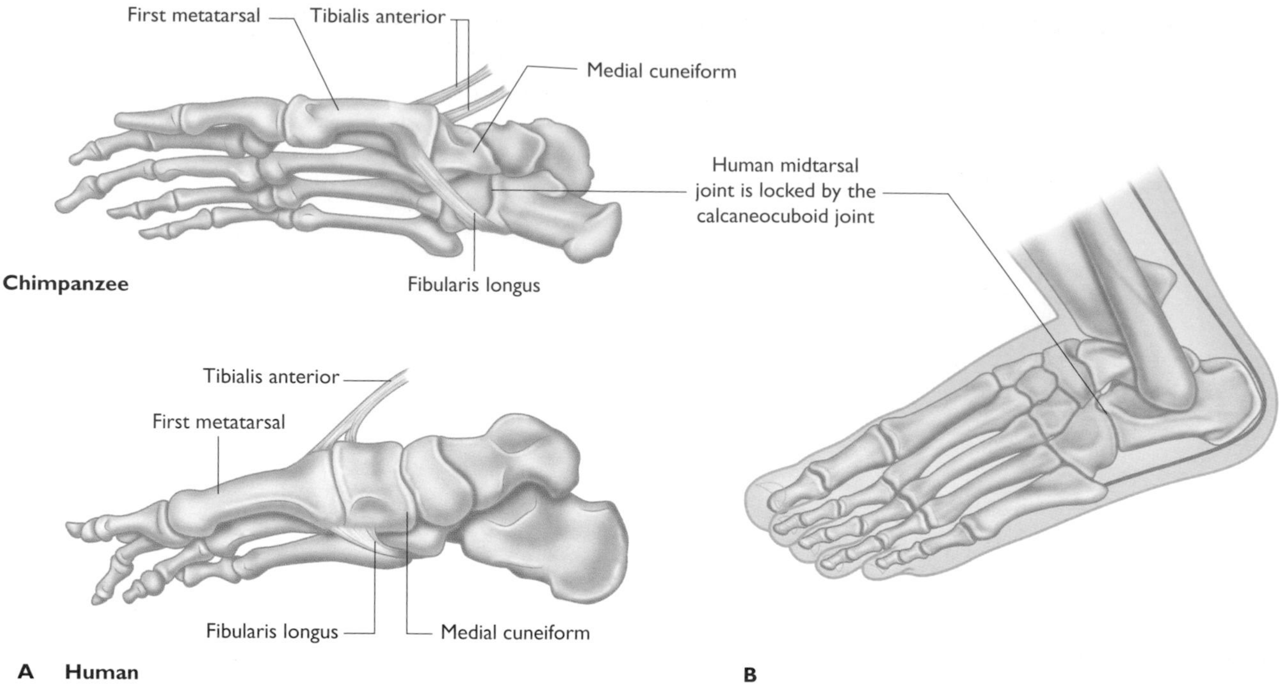

Figure 2.15.   A, The tibialis anterior and fibularis longus tendons attach to only the first metatarsal in contrast to those of the human, which attach to both the first metatarsal and the medial cuneiform. (Adapted from Conroy and Pontzer 2012.) B, The calcaneocuboid joint is slightly indented to allow the midtarsal line to lock and produce a rigid lever in the human foot.

feet fail to demonstrate the same capacity to produce the solid platform that humans use during toe-off. The grasping big toe of the nonhuman primates requires flexibility of the calcaneonavicular and calcaneocuboid joints, with each bone having separate muscle attachments for individual control (Conroy and Pontzer 2012; see fig. 2.15). For example, the chimpanzee tibialis anterior and fibularis longus tendons only attach to individual bones, while in the human foot they both attach to the first metatarsal as well the medial cuneiform (Aiello and Dean 2002). Having tendon attachments across adjacent bones reduces the independence of each bone and gives weaker fine control; however, this is less of an issue for the human foot, which has been repurposed toward efficient terrestrial walking and away from arborealism.

Reduced independence of the bones along the first ray of the human foot is not a bad thing—everything in biology is a compromise between associated costs and benefits. We may have lost mobility and range but we gained the stability of a rigid half-dome ready for toe-off. There are a number of structural elements within the design of the half-dome that provide the necessary stability. The first is the cuneiform arrangement of wedge-like bones that meet the equally wedged metatarsal bases (see fig. 2.10), and the second is another evolutionary adaptation within the calcaneocuboid joint, which has developed a projection to "lock" the midtarsal line as the foot supinates (fig. 2.15). Both of these structural elements give the foot some skeletal support, but they also require extra assistance from the soft tissues to create a symbiotic relationship between the skeletal and soft-tissue systems.

Form and Force Closure of the Foot

Form closure and *force closure* are terms more commonly associated with the sacroiliac joints (SIJs), but I find it useful to repurpose them when describing the combined hard- and soft-tissue strategies used by the foot during the rigid-mobile-rigid changes through the stance phase. *Form closure* refers to the natural support afforded by the arrangement and architecture of the bones and ligaments, while *force closure* is the extra support and stability provided by the muscles and tendons. In the case of the SIJ, the wedge arrangement of the bones gives some inherent support (form), which is assisted by the piriformis and the inferior portion of the gluteus maximus, which cross the joint (force).

The skeletal stability of the half-dome of the foot is supplied by the wedge-like cuneiforms and the locking of the midtarsal joint at the calcaneocuboid joint. However, we saw above that the form of the foot can unlock because of the offset between the talus and the calcaneus, especially following heel strike. The talocalcaneal offset acts as a key to unlock the foot and sets up a series of predictable reactions through the foot and into the rest of the lower limb. The downward glide of the talus on the sustentaculum talus creates a series of lateral rotations through the joints of the foot (see fig. 2.14*B*) and couples a series of medial rotations upward to the tibia, fibula, and femur.[3]

This "form opening" of the foot following heel strike allows the joints to open and the tissue to respond to the impact forces during the rest of early stance and mid-stance, but from mid-stance onward the foot must begin to recover its rigidity. After mid-stance, the swing leg comes in front of the body, pulling the pelvis in the direction of the stance foot and causes the femur on that side to laterally rotate. The tibia and fibula follow the lateral rotation of the femur above them and couple the lateral rotation down to the talus. The lateral rotation of the talus reverses the medial rotation performed during pronation and thereby encourages the bones of the foot to "form close" (see fig. 2.15*B*).

"Force closure" of the foot takes place between mid-stance and toe-off as the plantar tissues tension. As the ankle dorsiflexes, all of the plantar flexor muscles will contract to control

and decelerate the movement. These muscles will include the two fibulares, tibialis posterior, flexors hallucis, and digitorum longus, along with the soleus and gastrocnemius, which tension the plantar fascia via the Achilles' tendon (see fig. 2.16). Each of these muscles helps draw the bones together to close-pack them and assist the foot's stability as the heel begins to lift during late stance and into toe extension; this is a fragile phase because of the long lever that has been created between the point of support—the metatarsal heads—and the body weight being carried down through the talus.

As the heel continues to rise, the metatarsophalangeal joints extend and further tension the long and short toe flexors and the plantar fascia. The tensioning of the flexor hallucis longus is particularly important as this muscle spans the inside of the foot's half-dome and crosses below the sustentaculum talus (see fig. 2.16). The long tendon of the flexor hallucis longus helps to lift and support the previously tilted sustentaculum talus, but it can only do this effectively and easily if the big toe is able to extend; a loss of toe extension will reduce the tendon's ability to assist the correction of the calcaneus.

Tensioning soft tissue to support foot supination as described above is commonly referred to as the *windlass mechanism*, and various descriptions of this can be found in numerous texts. I have chosen not to use this term, as so few people know what a "windlass" is,[4] and so the name does not really help visualize the mechanism. My preference is to use the terms *form closure* and *force closure*, because they are easier to visualize; moreover, both mechanisms occur simultaneously as the lower limb moves in response to gravity,

---

[3] It might be useful to review this section again after studying the "Real and Relative Motion" section below.

[4] I had to look it up myself! A *windlass* is a system of pulleys, cranks, and cables used to lift heavy objects; it therefore appears to be an ideal descriptor for the tendons crossing the pulleys of the ankle and toe joints, if only it was a better-known system. For that reason, my preference is to refer to the *force closure* of the foot.

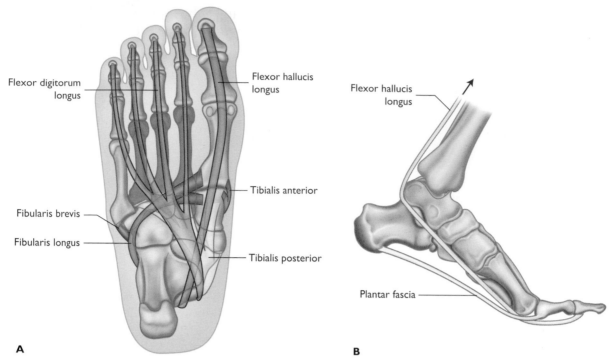

Figure 2.16.   A, All of the plantar flexors assist with force closure of the foot during ankle dorsiflexion. B, As the heel rises to create toe extension, the flexor hallucis longus tendon tensions to help support the inside of the foot's half-dome.

ground reaction force, and momentum, and the soft tissues (force) respond in accordance with the skeletal (form) dynamics.

The Joints and the Soft Tissue

It is the balance between mobility and stability—moving enough and not too much, and with the strength to control it—that defines healthy walking. The ability to first see any faults and then intervene with appropriate action is the role of the therapist. Therefore, as we build the picture of movement in each plane, we will also break it down into a series of "essential events"—the things that must occur in each joint to allow the myofascia to properly engage and perhaps communicate force across the various boney and soft-tissue interfaces.

As an easy example, consider the hamstrings: when the knee is extended, the tissues of the gastrocnemius and the hamstrings will interact with one another. One can feel this when performing a simple forward bend with the

knees extended; the range of motion is greatly increased, however, if the bend is done with the knees flexed, which disengages these tissues (see fig. 2.17).

Myofascial tissue, with its potential for continuity, can therefore provide us with a map of how the body can transfer mechanical force across body segments when the tissue is allowed to engage. This transfer and capture of force will require the correct amount of motion at each joint (the "essential events"). And, as we will see, myofascial tissue also provides us with the tracks through which mechanical information can travel. By following the vectors of force created by the interactions of gravity, ground reaction force, momentum, and joint alignment, we can easily see the contribution of the myofascial tissues to elastic efficiency, propulsion, stability, and shock absorption.

The multifaceted, three-dimensional fascial tissue uses shock absorption to stiffen and load the appropriate tissue along the various vectors of force following contact of the foot with the ground, and then it uses that stored energy to

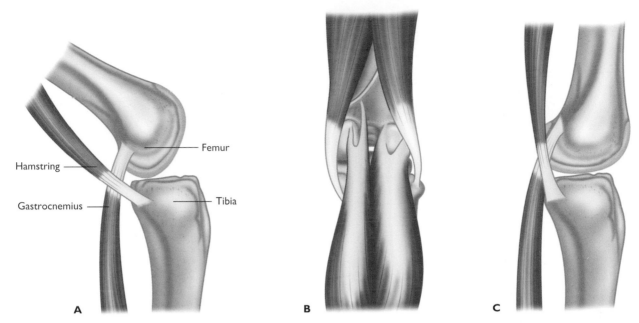

Hamstring
Gastrocnemius
Femur
Tibia

A   **B**   **C**

Figure 2.17. When the flexed knee joint (A) approaches the end of range (B and C), the tissue across the joint becomes aligned and allows the force from one segment to travel to the next. This dynamic can work in any direction, through each of the planes of motion. We will see that this is vital in the creation of myofascial elastic "triggers," which lead to the catapult effect, the release of elastic force to assist with propulsion (see chapter 3). Though the example shown here refers to the knee, the same principle will hold true in the body's other joints as well—to communicate force across the joints, they must achieve a certain degree of motion.

assist with propulsion in the opposite direction. In order to fully appreciate this, we must first analyze bone and joint movement during the gait cycle.

Joint Movement—Real and Relative

To build a clear understanding of tissue reactions during gait, we must be careful in the descriptive language we use. Many therapists and movement teachers confuse and conflate the movement of bones with the movement at the joints, and thereby create many difficulties in describing exactly what is taking place. It is worthwhile spending some time to clarify the two descriptive conventions of *arthrokinematics* and *osteokinematics*, which are so rarely used, despite providing a powerful tool for describing movement.

Being able to visualize soft-tissue actions and reactions during the gait cycle requires clarity of the sequence of adaptations of the bones and joints during the gait cycle. We will start with the foot and the most common place of first

interaction with the walking surface, the heel. There are two ways in which we can analyze the movement of the skeletal system: the *real movement* of the bones and the *relative movement* at the joints. For example, as we saw above, the tibia rotates medially after heel strike, and this will encourage the femur to rotate medially as well. These are the real movements of the bones. However, the amount of medial rotation of the two bones is not necessarily the same, and this creates a relative movement within the joint. If the tibia has moved further and faster than the femur, we would describe the knee as being medially rotated. The action at the joint will be determined by the *relative motion*, the amount by which one bone has moved in relation to the other. However, if the femur somehow medially rotated further and/or faster than the tibia, it would create a relative lateral rotation at the knee joint (see fig. 2.18).

These two methods of analyzing the movements of the skeletal system are also called *osteokinematic* (bone centered and "real," i.e., the actual movement of the bones in space) and *arthrokinematic* (joint centered,

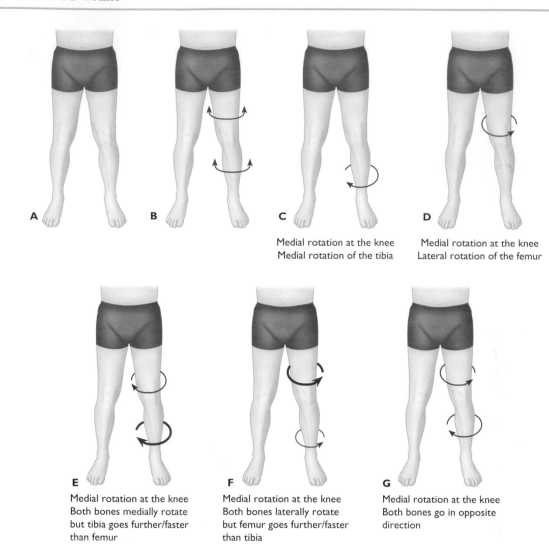

Medial rotation at the knee
Medial rotation of the tibia

Medial rotation at the knee
Lateral rotation of the femur

Medial rotation at the knee
Both bones medially rotate
but tibia goes further/faster
than femur

Medial rotation at the knee
Both bones laterally rotate
but femur goes further/faster
than tibia

Medial rotation at the knee
Both bones go in opposite
direction

Figure 2.18. *If we start with the two lower limb bones in neutral (A), we have six options for movement. If they both move in the same direction and at the same real speed (B), there is no relative change or motion at the joint. To create a relative medial rotation at the knee joint, we either medially rotate the tibia (C) or laterally rotate the femur (D). If both bones move medially, we can get the same medial rotation relationship across the joint by the tibia rotating further and/or faster than the femur (E). If both bones rotate laterally but the femur moves further/faster, relative medial rotation is created at the knee (F). If both bones go in opposite directions (G), the relative motion will be defined by the direction in which the distal bone moved. Note that the relationship at the joint is defined by the position of the distal bone in the body, except when referring to the spine, where it is the superior bone that defines the relationship.*

with the two bones moving relative to each other). To fully describe the events of gait, we will, at times, need to use both conventions to appreciate what is happening in the soft tissue.

Understanding the differences between real and relative motion is not just an academic exercise—it is important for our ability to see how strains are transferred across or through joints. We will see each of the possible variations leading to the same relative

movement at the joint strain the tissues in exactly the same vector, regardless of which of the real five motions described above (fig. 2.18C–F is used. As we saw above, strain across the talar joint creates the potential for coupling because of the overlap of the malleoli and the talus. Since the talar joint is relatively fixed in the transverse plane, the movement of one bone is almost directly coupled to the other. In the knee joint, however, there is no boney overlap, and coupling across this joint occurs via its associated soft tissues. Below we will appreciate the significance of the direction of soft-tissue strain.

Heel Strike and the Adaptation of the Foot

The foot's ability to deal with the ground reaction forces illustrated in figs. 2.13 & 2.19 is a primary determinant of the response through the body following heel strike. But, as we will see below, the foot requires assistance from the rest of the body to return to supination in preparation for toe-off. The first contact of the foot with the ground is perhaps the most important event in this chain. It is the first stage of the "stance" phase (see fig. 2.5 above), and it will define what happens throughout the rest of the body, provided the body can accept and adapt to this impact: tensegrity in action.

The ankle complex is only the first in a series of joints that should absorb some of the shock of impact. The knee and then the hip will be the next major shock absorbers, followed by the spine. It is therefore the accumulation of small corrections that both spread the load of the shock and stimulate the appropriate myofascial response.

With the foot in front of the body and the first contact coming to the heel, the ground reaction force will be angled posteriorly and superiorly, causing the ankle to plantar flex and decelerate (see fig. 2.20A).

Some writers have described the form of the back of the foot as a flawed design, because of the greater portion of body weight being transferred through the talus, which is not fully on top of the calcaneus (see fig. 2.20B); however, this arrangement is key to unlocking the foot's skeletal half-dome. As we saw earlier (fig. 2.14), this design is essential for the easy, economical, and shock-absorbing walking that we all aim for. On a firm surface, the calcaneus will be brought to an abrupt stop, but some of the body's momentum will still be bearing down on top of it. A significant portion of the weight

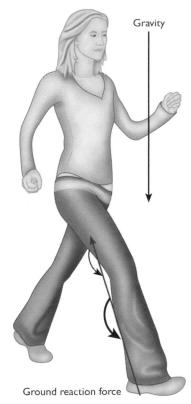

Figure 2.19. *Impact with the ground leads to a quick deceleration of the foot of the swing leg, and the interaction of the forward momentum of the foot and the ground reaction force will create a strong deceleration of the calcaneus.*

coming onto it is resting on the sustentaculum talus—a ledge of bone sometimes referred to as the *waiter's tray*—and this arrangement forces the calcaneus to tilt under the weight descending through the talus (see fig. 2.20B).

The tilt, or eversion, of the calcaneus (approximately 5 degrees) causes the talus to also tilt medially and to rotate medially. This movement within the subtalar joint affects the joints between the talus and both the navicular and the cuboid. Because of this, the more proximal tarsal bones will rotate more quickly, which will create a relative lateral rotation of the midtarsal joints (see fig. 2.21B). This movement of the metatarsal bones unlocks the midtarsal line and affords the foot more freedom to adapt to the potentially random ground surface. This relaxation of the "form closure" of the foot also assists in sending the shock to the thick plantar tissues, spreading the force more widely (see fig. 2.14C).

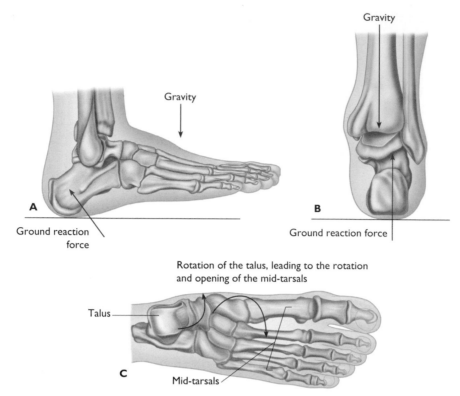

Figure 2.20. *At heel strike, the position of the calcaneus will act like one end of a see-saw and force the foot into a sudden plantar flexion (A), medially tilt the calcaneus, also referred to as "eversion" (B), and, finally, medially rotate the calcaneus—and therefore the talus and lower limb—as the talus slides down the offset sustentaculum talus (C).*

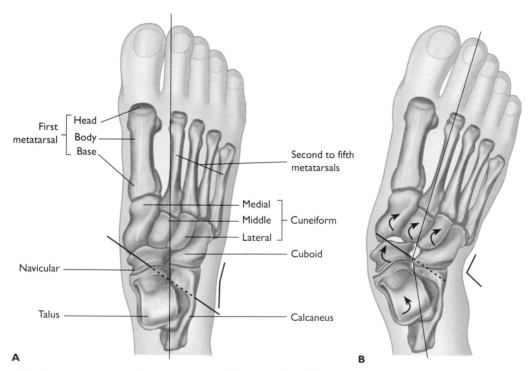

Figure 2.21. *Following heel strike, the calcaneus and talus of the neutral foot (A) will rotate medially (B). The navicular and cuboid follow more slowly and therefore create a relative lateral rotation at their joints with the talus. This unlocks the mid-tarsal joint and allows the tarsal bones to open and adapt to the ground.*

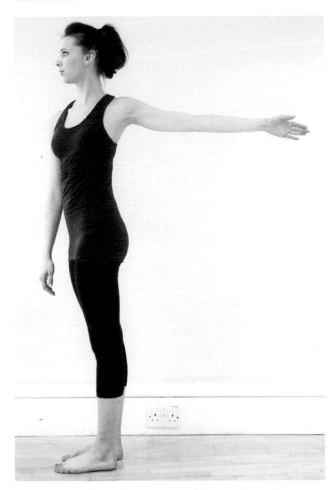

Figure 2.22. *Feeling the movement of the tarsal bones in exercise 2.1.*

Exercise 2.1. To feel the opening of the bones of the foot, stand with both feet quite close together and parallel. Bring one or both hands in front of you and turn as far as is comfortable to your left (as shown in fig. 2.22), keeping both feet on the ground. Be sure to allow your pelvis to move with you. Try to move the midtarsal bones within the right foot. Compare that sensation to the movement available on the left. You should feel more movement on the right, because the heel of that foot is more internally rotated, similar to the action at heel strike.

Weight Acceptance and the Adaptation of the Leg

Eversion of the calcaneus causes a medial rotation of the talus, which, in turn, causes a medial rotation of the tibia and fibula, since the talus is held in a mortise-and-tenon joint by the two leg bones (see fig. 2.23). The tibia and fibula medially rotate approximately 4 to 8 degrees as the knee flexes and comes across the front of the body, producing a valgus relationship at the knee joint (*valgus* refers to the angle created between the two bones forming the knee—in a valgus position, the tibia will angle down and out away from the femur, fig. 2.24).

The medial rotation of the tibia will also draw the femur into a medial rotation, but the tibia is moving faster and further than the femur. This means that the relative relationship between the two bones will be a medial rotation (of the tibia compared to the femur) at the knee. In the hip joint, the femur and pelvis are rotating in the same direction, but the pelvis will have rotated away from the swing leg during the stride, and the hip joint will therefore be laterally rotated.

After heel strike, as the weight is transferred to the lower limb, the knee will flex from its relatively straight angle at heel strike (by anything up to 20 degrees), and the hip will adduct (by approximately 4 to 5 degrees) as the pelvis receives the weight of the upper body (see fig. 2.25).

While most of the lateral tilt of the pelvis is lessened by the adaptation of the lumbars (detailed in chapter 4), the lumbars are much less able to reduce the rotation of the pelvis. The body has a number of mechanisms to contain rotation, the main one being the forward swing of the upper girdle on the opposite side, which helps rotate the upper thoracics in the opposite direction of the rotation of the pelvis. The rotation coming up from the pelvis and lower limbs therefore "meets" the counterrotation of the upper thoracics, and they cancel each other out before the movement reaches the neck and head (detailed in chapter 5, fig. 2.26).

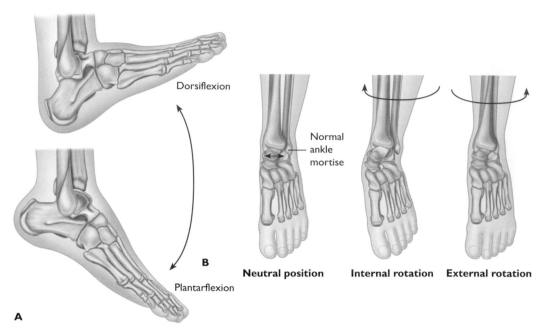

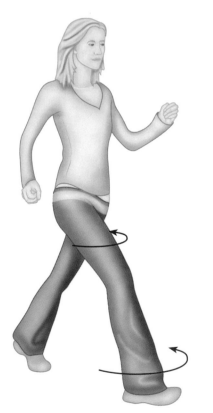

Dorsiflexion

Plantarflexion

A

Normal
ankle
mortise

Neutral position   **Internal rotation**   **External rotation**

B

Figure 2.23.   The mortise-and-tenon arrangement of the bones of the talar joint allows an independent motion of the foot in the sagittal plane of motion—plantar flexion and dorsiflexion (A). When a transverse motion is introduced, the three bones will follow each other, because of the security inherent in this type of joint (B). This is the cause of the difference of movement in the two feet in exercise 2.1. If you try the exercise again, you will sense that your right and left legs are internally and externally rotated, respectively. The rotation of the lower leg affects the positioning of the talus.

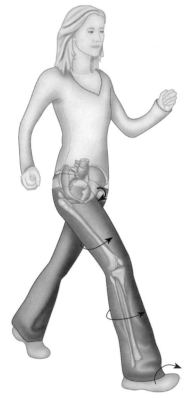

Figure 2.24.   As we progress up the leg, all of the bones are moving in the same direction (osteokinematics), and the relationship at the joints (arthrokinematics) is a medial rotation: the bones are all moving medially, but, because of the different speeds and degrees of movement, the inferior bone at each joint is medially rotated when compared to its superior neighbor.

Figure 2.25.   As the weight is passed to the forward limb, the knee flexes for additional shock absorption. Because the body's center of gravity is medial to the hip joint, the pelvis is encouraged into adduction as the laterally facing hip abductors receive the weight of the upper body and contract to keep it upright. This tilt of the pelvis has to be corrected in the spine before reaching the head—much of this is achieved by the lower three lumbar vertebrae.

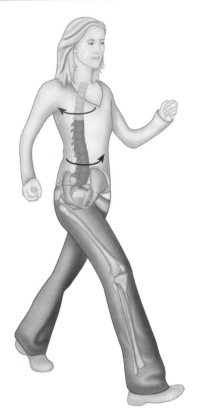

All of the above actions occur immediately following heel strike (0–2%) and as the foot receives the weight of the upper body (2–12%). The deceleration of the foot as it contacts the ground causes a roll on the calcaneus, plantar flexing the ankle. The foot, now firmly planted, cannot move further forward (unless walking on ice), so the momentum of the body forces the tibia and fibula to pivot over the talar joint, similar to a vaulter's pole. The pivot of the tibia and fibula brings the ankle through into dorsiflexion until the posterior tissues at the ankle reach the limit of their range of motion. At that point, the additional forward motion of the body will cause the foot to roll onto the ball of the foot (see fig. 2.27).

Note that as the heel rises to create the forefoot and toe rockers, a long lever is created between the ankle joint and the foot's distal point of contact. Body weight and some downward momentum will be pressing downward at the ankle while the forefoot is supporting the body. It is through these phases, from late stance to toe-off (31–62%), that we require extra stability in the foot. The form- and force-closure

Figure 2.26.   As the right foot heel strikes, the pelvis will be rotated to the left, which will also rotate the sacrum and the lumbars to the left. This is partly counterbalanced by the swing of the arms in the opposite direction, encouraging the upper thoracics to rotate to the right. These two rotational forces should balance each other out somewhere around T8.

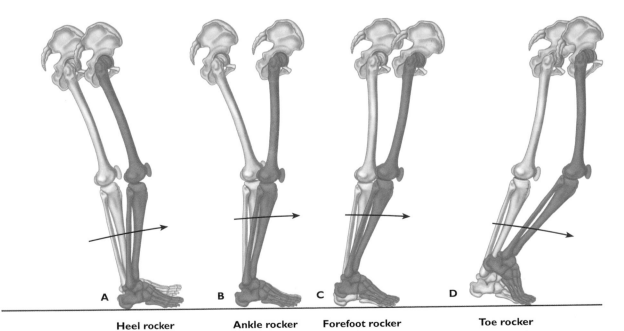

A   Heel rocker   **B**   Ankle rocker   **C**   Forefoot rocker   **D**   Toe rocker

Figure 2.27.   The four stages that lead to the toe-off for forward propulsion. The initial heel strike (A) and receiving of body weight cause the foot to brake, come into plantar flexion, and have full contact with the ground. This process causes the midtarsal joints to open and allows the foot to adapt with a slightly lowered arch, which also spreads the force of the impact to tissues deep to the plantar fascia. The swing of the opposite leg (B) and progress of the pelvis and trunk through space will cause the tibia and fibula to dorsiflex over the foot and then the heel to lift, creating a rocking motion on the ball of the foot (C), leading to the toe-off from the ends of the metatarsals and the toes (D).

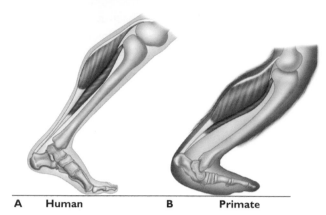

A   Human   B   Primate

Figure 2.28.   The benefit of the locking mechanism in the human midtarsal joint (B) is the ability to create a rigid lever during the latter stages of the stance phase in preparation for toe-off. The nonhuman primate foot (A) remains in contact with the ground for longer because of the midtarsal break (the ability to left the heel independently of the rest of the foot).

mechanisms must occur in order to recover the foot's skeletal integrity, otherwise the soft tissue may have to compensate by carrying the extra stress (see fig. 2.28).

The swing of the opposite leg drives the correction of the rotations that occurred following heel strike. As the swing leg comes through from posterior to anterior, it will, by necessity, turn the pelvis in the opposite direction. The movement of the pelvis will then laterally rotate the femur of the planted leg, which will rotate the tibia and fibula, and they in turn will rotate the talus and therefore the calcaneus.

This brings us back to the pronation and supination felt in exercise 2.1. The bones of the foot on the medially rotating limb are in a loose and adaptable form, while those of the laterally rotating limb are much more solid, stable, and compact. We need the correction back to an integrated, stable foot to prepare for the increased forces experienced at toe-off. The loose foot, ideal for molding to the impact surface during the early stance phase, becomes a more solid foot for rolling forward onto the ball of the foot prior to toe-off (see fig. 2.29).

The re-supination of the foot is driven by the two closure dynamics. The relative dorsiflexion

and eventual toe extension tension the plantar flexors and toe flexors to give force closure, while the lateral rotation of the talus creates form closure. The lateral rotation of the bones of the stance leg is driven by the rotation of the pelvis in response to the swing leg. In this case, the pelvis turns more than the femur, which creates the medial rotation at the hip and, because the femur turns more than the tibia, medial rotation is also created across the knee.

It is worth spending a little time to clarify the relative motions of the joints, as it helps us visualize what is happening in the soft tissues. Following heel strike, the medial rotations are driven upward from the tilt of the calcaneus, and the tibia therefore rotates medially further than the femur, which is easy to see as "medial rotation at the knee." However, during the late stance phase, as the other leg swings through and the pelvis turns, the lateral rotation of the bones is driven downward from the pelvis to the femur to the tibia and to the talus, which means the superior bones turn further than the inferior bones. If we return to fig. 2.7 for reference, we can see that if both bones turn medially but the inferior one turns further, a medial rotation occurs at the knee, and if both bones turn laterally but the superior one turns further, a medial rotation is also created at the knee.

The significance of this becomes clearer on observing the arrangement of the cruciate ligaments of the knee. Although they are better known for assisting anterior-posterior stability of the knee joint, the cruciate ligaments lie in an oblique angle in the transverse plane (see fig. 2.30). Their obliquity is such that they couple medial rotation of the knee, and they are uncoupled during lateral rotation of the knee. Words can get in the way of being able to see the significance of the relationship and the coupling, but if we look at the angle of movement in which the cruciate ligaments couple motion (fig 2.30D), it can be easier to visualize that turning the femur laterally will pull the tibia, and pulling the tibia medially will also pull the femur.

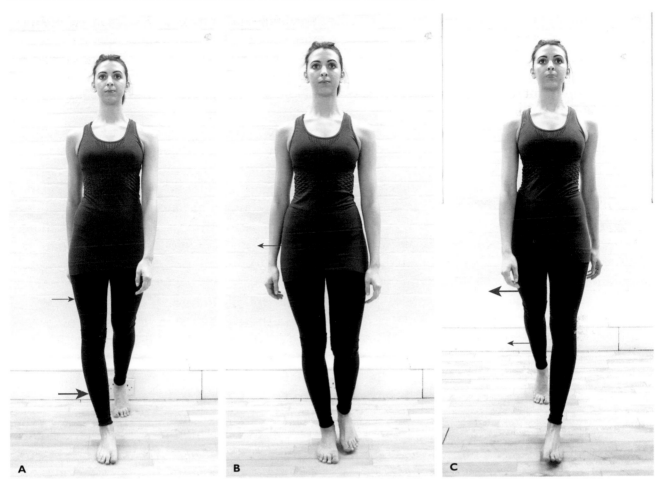

Figure 2.29. *The rotation is determined by what is moving fastest at any one time. At the moment of heel strike, it is the eversion of the calcaneus that determines the chain of events upward into the rest of the body. Once the forward foot is planted on the ground (A), the back leg will then be accelerating from its toe-off, and its momentum and anterior reach will turn the pelvis to the opposite side, creating a correcting rotation through the forward leg (B and C).*

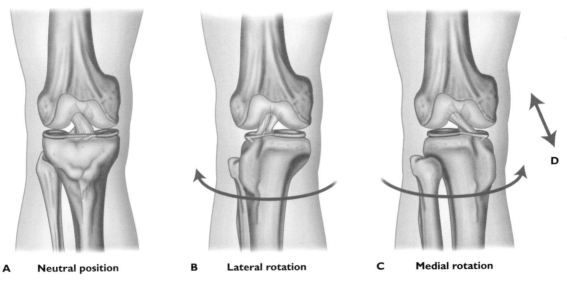

| A | Neutral position | B | Lateral rotation | C | Medial rotation |

Figure 2.30. *The cruciate ligaments of the knee (A) unlock during lateral rotation of the knee (B) and lock during medial rotation (C). There are five possible ways of creating the relative motion of medial rotation at the knee—we need to refer back to fig. 2.18C–F. It can sometimes be easier to see the vector of force (D) passing through the knee tissue, resulting from movement of the tibia, femur, or both bones in the various combinations.*

The re-supination of the foot benefits from form closure for extra stability, and the form closure of the foot is driven by the lateral rotations of the bones above it. The swing leg therefore plays an important role in the re-supination of the stance foot, but that role can only be successful because of the coupling mechanism across the knee.

The Rest of the Body

The upper body will also continuously adapt through the gait cycle. The movement and angulation of the pelvis and the swing of the arms are two of the keys for understanding the body's movement. Any movement created in the lower body will have to be diminished before it reaches the head, in order for the eyes to remain steady and for the brain not to be traumatized by heel strike. The arms are used to counterbalance the forces going to the head in each of the planes of movement; however, they also contribute to the elastic forces acting through the trunk, especially in oblique planes, and each arm works with the movement of the opposite lower limb. While the upper body makes a significant contribution to walking, its actions are somewhat more straightforward and will be discussed later.

■ MOVING FORWARD

The main focus of the next few chapters will be an analysis of the positions of the body at the two extremes: heel strike (including the process of weight acceptance) and toe-off. It is at these points that the soft tissue is most engaged, stretched across the joints, and carrying more force, as the point of contact with the ground will be further from the body's center of gravity.

At heel strike and toe-off, the tissue is preparing for the various reactions determined by joint alignment through the rest of the body. By first understanding the pattern created in

the bones and joints, we can look at where the force of impact is directed to in the soft tissues. We can see how the skeletal mechanics are detected by the proprioceptive system in the myofascia, which alert the appropriate muscles to decelerate downward movement of the body caused by the interaction of momentum, gravity, and ground reaction force. With this mechanism of deceleration in place, the body can reverse the sequencing of the chain with maximum efficiency, by using all of the elements of the stretch-shortening cycle and fascial recoil that allow walking to be energy efficient, easy, and graceful.

It is the folding of the joints that creates the prestress—the countermovement or preparatory movement—that stimulates muscle spindles and mechanoreceptors to initiate an isometric contraction. That tightening of the muscles allows the associated fascia to absorb any further deceleration force. Once the fascia is at its elastic transition point, it can recoil like a spring. Furthermore, any requisite concentric contraction of the muscle is made more powerful as it pushes against the taut surrounding bag of tissues—the combined epimysium, endomysium, and perimysium.

If there is a fault in this system—if one joint movement is missing or restricted—muscle fibers somewhere along the chain may not be switched on, causing others to compensate. We recognize the fault when we feel we must make a special effort to continue moving. The next chapters will trace in more detail the important events in the joints that enhance the tissues' abilities to function with elastic kinetic energy along each plane.

■ SUMMARY

1. There are four main functions of walking—propulsion, stance stability, energy conservation, and shock absorption.

2. When putting the skeletal system and its joint alignment into context of the gait cycle, we can build a picture of the soft-tissue response.

3. Insights into different movement strategies can be gleaned from comparative and evolutionary anatomy, which assumes a drive toward increased efficiency and economy of movement.

4. Evolutionary skeletal changes, especially in the foot and spine, facilitate longer strides and allow more tissues to be strained by momentum as the body moves forward.

5. A long stride requires toe extension, hip extension, and lumbar extension, and these ranges of motion allow the fascial tissues to capture energy involved in momentum.

6. Offsets between ground reaction force and center of gravity, such as between the sustentaculum talus and the talus and at the lateral hip, can also be used to stiffen the tissues to take advantage of pre-tensioning dynamics in the soft tissues.

7. The human foot has become specialized to deliver both a mobile adaptor for heel strike and weight acceptance and a rigid lever in preparation for toe-off. The foot's function is best described using the ideas of form and force closure.

8. Osteokinematics and arthrokinematics provide necessary clarity to describe movement of the bone (*osteo*/real motion) or at the joint (*arthro*/relative).

3

SAGITTAL PLANE

You cannot teach a crab to walk straight.

—Aristophanes

■ INTRODUCTION

Walking straight ahead is our default, but not everyone actually accomplishes this all of the time. Deviations occur for a number of reasons that we investigate later in this chapter. Sagittal plane progression requires flexion and extension, which are probably the most obvious movements we see in walking and have formed the basis of most gait analyses.

Unlike our crustacean friends, our predominant joint movement[1] below the hip is in the sagittal plane with the movements of flexion and extension. It is the in-series alignment of joints that determines much of our movement strategy and allows us to "walk straight."

That is not to say important elements of the frontal and transverse planes are not present, but they will be dealt with in chapters 4 and 5, respectively, as we build up the fuller, more authentic, three-dimensional image in further chapters.

Our ability to move forward uses extension through the whole body, and we will see how extension stiffens many tissues whose various degrees of fascial continuity and connection all cooperate to control momentum and recycle the energy for the swing phase. However, the ability to use sagittal plane progression to appropriately load the tissues requires the following essential events:

- Each of the foot rockers—heel, ankle, forefoot, and toe
- Knee extension
- Hip extension
- Lumbar, thoracic, and cervical extension

The two main models of gait, the inverted pendulum and the spring-mass system, were introduced in chapter 1 (see fig. 1.8). As we saw, the inverted pendulum model cannot work without soft tissue to catch its tick-tock action as the hip flexes and extends. The spring-mass system matches the forces more closely, as the pelvis needs to be efficiently caught by the elastic tissue either side of the

---

[1]The knee, talar joint, and metatarsophalangeal joints all have relatively large ranges of motion in the sagittal plane, especially compared to the many smaller joints of the foot. These small joints may move in other planes, but their range is not as large; they are still important but they contribute less to the length of stride.

hip joints. The fall and rise of the pelvis will be explored in the next chapter, as our focus for this chapter will be the events that ensure optimal loading of the flexor and extensor tissues. Optimal loading benefits from a long stride length, as it positively affects the pre-tensioning of the myofascial tissues and allows elastic energy to be captured by them. As we will see below, there are many interdependent events that can negatively affect sagittal plane progression and shorten the stride, or create compensations that exaggerate movement in either of the two other planes.

A Note on the Use of Planes

I feel we must address the elephant in the room by acknowledging that there is no such thing as sagittal, frontal, and transverse plane movement—there is just *movement*—and movement happens in all three planes *all* of the time. The use of planes is a construct that facilitates the description, and thereby the analysis, of the three-dimensional complexities of movement. To just say that everything is a spiral or everything "just moves" does not empower our exploration of what is going on and why. The three planes provide a coordinate system that describes position and action for anatomy, just as longitude and latitude serve a similar function for navigation. There are no actual lines on the Earth, but longitude and latitude give us a convention to know where we are, where "somewhere else" is, and how to get from here to there; the three planes of motion give us a similar power for describing the anatomy of movement. The use of planes becomes especially accurate when combined with an understanding of real and relative motion. With both conventions—planes and kinematics—in place, we can describe with clarity where we started a movement, where we ended up, and how we got there.

I should also point out that there is no such thing as a purely sagittal movement, and we could instead use the term *parasagittal*—or,

"close enough to sagittal." To avoid more jargon and to be consistent with other texts, I have chosen to use *sagittal* in the loose sense of "straight ahead."

It is also important to say that all muscles work in each plane to give extra support or add an essential line of support to help correct or control movement, but most have a predominant fiber direction to help control a movement vector at particular phases.

■ GETTING STARTED—I—WITH SAGITTAL LOADING

Before the body can concern itself with any of the phases of gait, it must first get started. As anyone who has worked with patients or a family member with neurological issues will attest, the initiation of gait can be difficult and frustrating. Initiation of gait is complex, and a number of mechanisms have to be in place to actually start walking. A full exploration of these mechanisms is beyond the remit of this text, but it is informative to analyze the work of Dalton, Bishop, Tillman, and Haas (2011), who demonstrated that placing the swing foot slightly behind the stance foot prior to taking the first step can increase forward propulsion and decrease the amount of time required for starting the step. This was found to be effective even if the swing foot was placed only half a foot behind the stance foot, which extends the hip and dorsiflexes the ankle. This simple repositioning was successful for both older adults and those diagnosed with Parkinson's disease, and it can be easily explained by the pre-tensioning of the tissue within the hip flexors as well as the plantar flexors of the foot and ankle.

Exercise 3.1. **One can quite easily feel the positive effect of the pre-tensioning of the front of the body by tapping your toe on the floor behind you. Try this by reaching back quite quickly with one foot to touch the floor behind you and then relaxing, trying not to** actively bring your leg back to its starting position. It will come back of its own volition, using the energy that has been put into the anterior tissue by the posterior swing of the leg, stretching its elastic elements. You may need to experiment a little before really getting the sense of it, but try at various speeds and with different amounts of force, and also try increasing the amount of time you allow the toe to stay on the floor behind you. Most people feel that increasing the speed increases the recoil, as does a longer range of motion, but only as far as you can go before the other hip has to flex, which compromises the continuity of the front of the body. Timing is also crucial—spend too long with your toe on the floor behind you, and you lose the momentum. This is the *amortization effect*: too long a pause, and much of the elastic loading is lost, wasted as heat and causing an increase in active work to return the leg forward again.

Exercise 3.1 gives us a possible explanation of why the Dalton experiment found a positive result from displacing the swing foot. Even a slight pre-tension within the tissue will lessen the amount of muscle work and coordination necessary to begin leg swing. The leg extension has provided elastic potential energy that can be used for the returning flexion.[2]

Preloading a tissue removes any slack from the fascial elements—it "shrink wraps" the fascia around the muscle—which means that once the muscles contained within the fascia are required to contract, the force created by the muscles is immediately transferred through the fascia's length. As we saw in chapter one, preloading the tissue effectively reduces the work required of the muscles and increases their relative power.

---

[2]It is called *potential energy* because it has not yet been used; it can be converted into other events. In the case of elastic energy, the potential produced is generally for movement in the opposite direction.

Myofascial Continuities, Anatomy Trains, or Lines of Tension?

The body's position at the end of the toe reach in exercise 3.1 mimics the position at toe-off when forward momentum, channeled through the joints, creates pre-tensioning along the anterior tissues. Try repeating the exercise with an anterior head position, with your rib cage in various tilts or shifts, and with your arms and shoulders in protraction and retraction. Each of these will influence the amount of "spring" you feel in the hip and may therefore need to be addressed in a client with compromised gait efficiency (see "Clinical Note" below).

The idea of the Superficial and Deep Front Lines (SFL and DFL; fig. 3.1A and B) from the Anatomy Trains model, used in the first edition of this text, give food for thought on the implications of structural and functional positioning of the upper body while walking. However, the reality of many of the connections proposed within the Anatomy Trains model has been called into question (Wilke et al. 2015), with especially little support shown for the SFL within the wider anatomical literature. Regardless of the continuity, from a functional point of view the actual connections are of less significance than the lines of tension made through the body during movement. Analyzing the production of tension along the sagittal plane is the primary focus of this chapter, as the extension through the body encourages the communication of force from one soft-tissue structure to another.

There are at least three ways in which force can be communicated between soft-tissue structures:

- Directly through fascial tissue as per the posterior oblique line consisting of the latissimus dorsi, thoracolumbar fascia, and gluteus maximus (Carvalhais et al. 2013; van Wingerden et al. 1993).

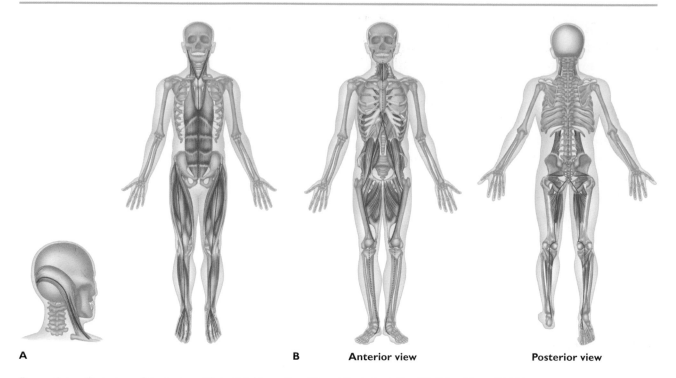

A   **B**   **Anterior view**   **Posterior view**

Figure 3.1. Illustration of the proposed Superficial Front Line (A) and Deep Front Line (B). (After Myers 2015.)

- Via the bone's elasticity (van Wingerden et al. 1993).
- Through the bone, regardless of the bone's elasticity and ability to deform under load (Myers 2015; see fig. 3.2).

It should be noted that the presence of myofascial continuity between structures does not necessarily imply the transmission of force. Myofascia can be continuous from one muscle to another but still be unable to communicate

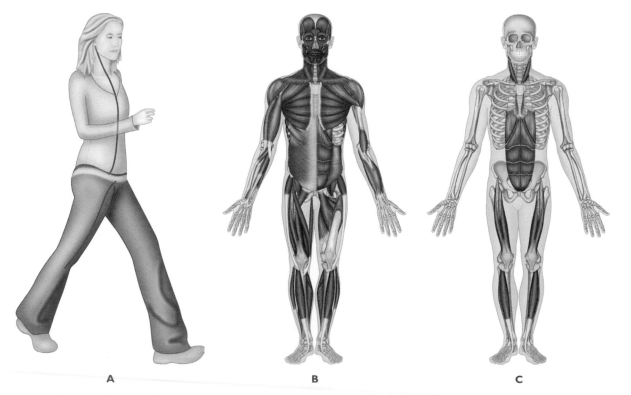

A   **B**   **C**

Figure 3.2. The toe-off position should pre-tension most of the anterior aspect of the body (A). If we focus our attention on the sagittal plane extension and remove soft tissues oriented in other planes (B), the Superficial Front Line is revealed but many more tissues will also be tensioned in this position (C).

(Schleip 2019, private communication). We must acknowledge anatomical variation in the amount of continuity and tissue stiffness, rather than making global assumptions of how force is transferred for each individual (van Wingerden et al. 1993).

In many cases the body does not necessarily require continuity and may actually benefit from a lack of transfer of force across attachments, something we will see in the next chapter with the stabilization of the pelvis in the frontal plane. If we consider the body as a tensegrity structure, the tensioning of tissue above and below a boney attachment will increase the bone's stability.[3] Stabilizing the bone will allow it to communicate in response to movement and act as a stiffer element (relative to the slightly less stiff tendons and the much less stiff myofascia) within the movement system. Myers' rationale for the break in continuity of the SFL between the rectus femoris and the rectus abdominis is that the pelvis can act as a rigid, stiff element to transfer force between these two muscles. Simply put, because of the stiffness of the pelvis, the rectus abdominis and rectus femoris do not have to be continuous with one another; these muscles are in opposition across the pelvis—pulling on one will affect the other.

The forces acting on the bone will be described by an equation based on gravity, momentum, and ground reaction balanced against the strength, mobility, and relative stiffnesses of the soft tissues attaching to the bone. Being able to visualize predominant tissue directions alongside these forces will allow you to understand the functional overlap between muscle fiber direction and movement direction, such as the body's extension at toe-off, which aligns with the flexor tissues. Gradually, as we build up the picture, I hope the reader will appreciate the body as an interrelated,

interactive whole, with the ability to adjust its stiffness in response to forces acting through it. When all of the pieces of the puzzle are in place, the question of tissue continuity becomes less important than the cooperative alliance between joint range, muscle fiber direction, and our common movement patterns.

Most of our movement happens in long chains; it is only on occasion at the gym or during an orthopedic test that we deliberately isolate certain joints and tissues. The overlap between movement patterns and soft-tissue arrangement is not accidental: they have to coexist—and this is something that has been noticed by many anatomists. The commonly taught Anatomy Trains model is a starting point to see the overlap between form and function, and it was a useful one for me—the reader must remember it is a simplification of the much more complex reality.

For example, studies have shown that many passive elastic tissues (fascial tissue of single- and two-joint muscles, joint capsule, ligament, and skin) are involved in up to 40 percent of the negative work required during hip extension (negative work is the deceleration of the movement; Silder et al. 2007). Once suitably loaded with potential energy, these tissues then provide approximately 50 percent of the net positive work during toe-off and initial swing (positive work is the return into flexion), which in this case is assisted by collagenous tissues on many tissue levels (Whittington et al. 2008). As we will see in the next chapter, limiting our vision to the tissues listed in any one anatomy model results in missing other important factors, and so we will widen our vision beyond single tissue layers.

The reality of the situation is that the body simultaneously uses a combination of mechanisms:

1. In-series pre-tensioning when force is transferred between myofascial units, as described by Vleeming and Myers.

---

[3]In the context of movement, the stability of a bone does not mean no movement but something closer to the sense of "controlled"—the bone is able to respond appropriately because of the balance of forces around it.

2. In-parallel pre-tensioning when force is transferred between layers, such as described in the hydraulic amplifier effect of the thigh (see chapter 4).

Clinical Note

Is the tensioning of the anterior tissue part of the reason for your client's posterior tilt of the rib cage? If the head is held in an anterior position it can shorten or reduce the stiffness of the anterior tissue (see fig. 3.3A), and the posterior tilt of the thorax is a common compensation (see fig. 3.3B). The posterior tilt of the thorax predominantly acts as a counterbalance to the acquired head position, but it may also assist with the tension created at the front of the body to help the recoil into flexion during gait.

■ SAGITTAL PLANE GAIT CYCLE

In the sagittal plane, toe-off is probably the most interesting part of the gait cycle because of the way it determines how much extension—and therefore how much tissue pre-tension—is achieved prior to the release of the leg into the swing phase. The appropriate pre-tensioning achieved in the extended position shown in fig. 3.2 determines much of the ease during the swing, as the release at toe-off should be an ideal blend of release of elastic energy and minimal concentric muscle contraction. We saw the advantage of sagittal pre-tension for those with neurological deficits earlier, but all of us can create similar advantages for each step by ensuring an appropriate stride length.

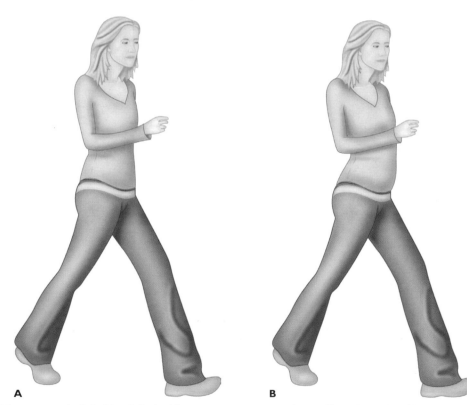

A   B

Figure 3.3. With an anteriorly shifted head, the body's anterior tissue may not be as effectively tensioned by hip extension (A), and this may be compensated for by posteriorly tilting the rib cage (B). In this way, both anterior and posterior tissues may develop areas of restriction as the body tries to create a certain kind of balance.

■ A WORD ON THE INTERPRETATION OF ELECTROMYOGRAPHY

Electromyography (EMG) records muscle activation by detecting the electric potential of muscle cells when the cells are activated. The scale used in the charts in fig. 3.4 is a percentage of *maximum voluntary contraction*, which allows us to see how hard the muscle may be working relative to its potential at any one phase.

There are a few limitations on the use of EMG for something as complex as gait: it does not give us a sense of the direction in which the muscle may be working (except by extrapolation, which we will have to do later on), and not every muscle has been measured during gait, giving us limited data to work from.

A major advantage of EMG readings, however, is that they let us see the actual function of muscles and expose how they often work in reverse of the traditionally described anatomical "action." Taking a measurement when a muscle is actually firing is necessary, because there is much confusion in the analysis of movement, especially gait. For example, some schools of thought teach that the gluteus maximus extends the hip during toe-off. However, a quick glance at the EMG chart in fig. 3.4 will show that the gluteus maximus is only active shortly before heel strike (95%) through to mid-stance (12%), and that it is quiescent from mid-stance onward, when the hip is extended. The gluteus maximus does not extend the hip; rather, it works to prevent further hip flexion when the hip is flexed and a long lever moment is present following heel strike.

The EMG readings also show that the rectus femoris is mostly active before toe-off, in those last few moments of hip extension and the first few degrees of flexion—a mixed pattern, but one that makes sense in terms of the control and deceleration of movement. Those last few degrees of hip extension prior to toe-off are also functionally significant, as we saw in the exercises above. If we lose toe extension, knee extension, or even lumbar extension, we are unlikely to reach the end of range in the hip and will therefore lose the contribution from the rectus femoris in the stance-to-swing transition.

It is also interesting to note the anatomical differences between the rectus femoris and the other quadriceps. The rectus femoris is on a different fascial layer from that of the other quadriceps (Nene et al. 2002), and is also pennate toward the hip, indicating its potential focus on hip rather than knee extension.

If we analyze the rectus femoris in the light of the nature of the ankle plantar flexors, we may get a better insight into the role of both. The pennation angle of the plantar flexors is consistently toward the ankle joint—the joint they are controlling. Therefore, does the rectus femoris, with its fibers angling medially and superiorly, play more of a role in deceleration of the hip joint than in knee extension? The existence of the rectus femoris on a separate fascial plane to that of the other quadriceps facilitates an independent glide of the muscle and gives it the freedom necessary to serve the hip.

The plantar flexors' role in controlling the foot and ankle is illustrated by the timings of the EMG readings. As the hip passes sagittal plane neutral at mid-stance (12%), forward momentum takes over and the ankle plantar flexors (see fig. 3.5—soleus, gastrocnemius, tibialis posterior, flexors hallucis and digitorum longus, and fibularis longus and brevis) tension to decelerate and control the ankle as it dorsiflexes and then the toes as they extend.

The EMG readings for the hamstring group (biceps femoris, semitendinosus, and semimembranosus) are also interesting, as these muscles begin to fire during mid-swing as the hip is flexing, once again showing that the same muscle is required to control the opposite

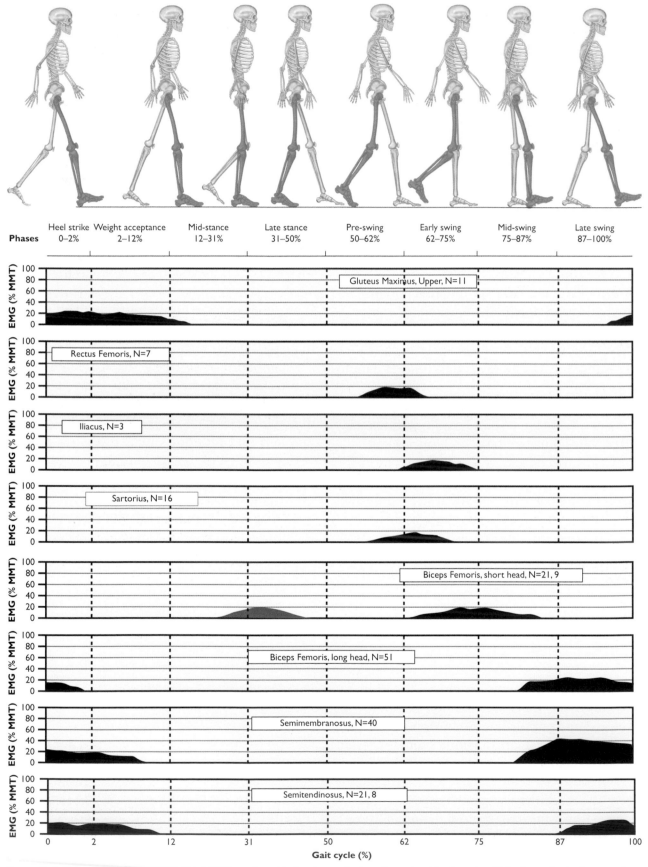

Figure 3.4. *The gait cycle and the related EMG readings. Notice the tensioning of muscle while the related joint is moving in the opposite direction of the muscle "action." (N = number of subjects measured.) (Adapted from Perry and Burnfield 2010.)*

movement of its "action." The hamstrings continue to contract through to mid-stance, and, similarly to gluteus maximus, they switch off when the hip begins to go into extension.

The apparent reversal of muscle contraction can be confusing if one adheres to the *actions* repeated in every textbook. Textbooks use an idealized world of open-chain, gravity- and momentum-free movement that often inhibits learning true muscle function, which is very flexible and context dependent. For example, one has to question whether the muscle is initiating movement (concentric contraction), decelerating a movement (eccentric), or working with the external forces of momentum and gravity along with ground reaction force (which could require any combination of concentric, eccentric, or isometric contraction, depending on the balance of the forces and on the possible need to adjust speed).

■ TOE-OFF AND PRE-SWING PHASE

I have chosen to use the term *toe-off* for what is commonly referred to as *push-off*, as the latter gives the impression of an active *push* from the plantar flexors. Push-off suggests concentric contraction, but the reality is more complex yet more efficient in terms of metabolic cost through the symbiosis of muscle, fascial tissue, and momentum.

Numerous researchers have found that when the body is experiencing rhythmical repeated movement, the system optimizes itself to reduce the work associated with concentric and eccentric contractions, and the muscle fibers remain relatively isometric. The muscles may be tensioning, but that does not necessarily mean that the fibers are shortening or lengthening; they are simply adjusting the stiffness in the tissues to optimize the capture and release of elastic energy through the use of momentum (Fukunaga et al. 2002; Sawicki et al. 2009; Robert 2016). As we saw in chapter 1, when combined with momentum, muscle force

will further strain (lengthen) the tendons, and the strain provides stored potential energy which can be utilized as kinetic energy in the return movement.

It is often quoted that tendons can strain to about 5 percent of their length and are extremely efficient at returning energy, giving back 97 percent of the energy used to stretch them (Alexander 2002). However, it is important to remember that, as Silder et al. (2007) proved, tissues other than just the tendons are involved in elastic mechanisms. When momentum is present in the system, all collagenous tissues have some ability to recycle kinetic energy—just to differing degrees and depending on their constituent levels of collagen fibers.

The release from the open extended position of toe-off to early swing should therefore represent a release of captured energy, rather than concentric muscle work pulling or pushing the body forward. The capture of kinetic energy requires enough momentum and enough range at each joint to allow the tissues to strain. There are a number of interdependencies between the joints when we go into movement, which I refer to, in the gait cycle, as the *essential events*. We will explore these essential event interdependencies as we progress through the phases and events of the gait cycle, especially in the build-up to the catapult and trigger-type mechanism seen at toe-off.

■ FOOT ROCKERS, FORCE CLOSURE, A CATAPULT

Walking is good for solving problems—it's like the feet are little psychiatrists.

—Pepper Giardino

As we saw in chapter 2 (see fig. 2.13), the foot must serve many functions during the stance phase as it progresses from being stable to mobile and back to forming a rigid lever again prior to toe-off. Each of those functions occurs during a different period with different joint relationships and therefore different tissue tensions. The stance period is commonly broken down into five separate phases (heel strike, weight acceptance, mid-stance, late stance, and pre-swing), during which time the foot and ankle progress through four so-called "rockers"—heel, ankle, forefoot, and toe. As we will see below, each rocker is an important event in itself for the adaptation of the foot, but they also relate to the swing and progress of the other foot and lower limb—the body is a truly interdependent entity.

Once the heel comes in contact with the floor, ground reaction force, interacting with gravity and with momentum from the body, causes the foot to roll on the calcaneus (see fig. 3.5)—the heel rocker. This use of forces is similar to that of a pole vaulter planting the pole and changing the downward movement of the pole into forward and upward movement. The interaction of the calcaneus and the ground forms a braking mechanism, encouraging the "pole" of the leg to pass above it.

As the pelvis progresses over the planted foot, the ankle joint changes from being plantar flexed to dorsiflexed—the ankle rocker. Eventually the ankle reaches the limit of its range, causing the heel to lift and the foot to rock onto the metatarsal heads and then quickly onto the toes—the forefoot and toe rockers.

For smooth progression through each of the four rockers, the joints must be free and the plantar flexors long enough to allow the full movement to occur. The tendons passing around the medial and lateral malleoli also have to be in balance to allow the foot to come back from the eversion/pronation created by heel strike and weight acceptance.

When we analyze the rockers alongside the EMG readings (fig. 3.5), the roles of the muscles become more obvious. All of the plantar flexors (soleus, gastrocnemius, tibialis posterior, flexor digitorum longus, flexor hallucis longus, fibularis longus, and fibularis brevis) are active to varying degrees between heel strike (0%) and toe-off (62%), as they act to control and decelerate the progression over the top of the foot—i.e., they are initially decelerating ankle dorsiflexion and then toe extension. It is through the deceleration of the "vault" over the foot that the kinetic energy from the body's momentum is captured by the plantar flexors and the anterior tissues above the thigh. The plantar flexors' function during these phases of gait can be visualized by imagining them as a series of elastic bands that lengthen in the passage from heel strike to toe-off.

The elastic tissues in the body vary in their stiffness and momentum, and will also change as a function of the speed of gait. Muscles therefore have to act as the instantaneous adjusters of tension and stiffness in the midst of this very complex interaction between constantly changing variables. We have seen that eccentric and concentric contractions are metabolically more expensive than isometric contractions, and that the muscles consume more energy when walking occurs beyond the "preferred transition speed"[4] (Shih et al. 2016; see also horse style transitions in fig. 1.29). The work of Sawicki and colleagues (2009) indicates that muscle tension will minimize energy use by optimizing toward isometric contraction. However, changes in muscle tension occur around the ankle complex as the body moves over the foot, and the muscle fibers "tune" the stiffness of the system by contracting concentrically, isometrically, or eccentrically in response to momentum and in context with the natural tendon stiffness. The muscle tension in the surrounding tissues acts as a "stiffness-adjusting system." If there is too much or not enough momentum, the muscles have to

---

[4]*Preferred transition speed* is the speed at which animals change their gait pattern, such as from a walk to a run. Walking slowly or quickly affects elastic loading and requires increased muscle adjustment.

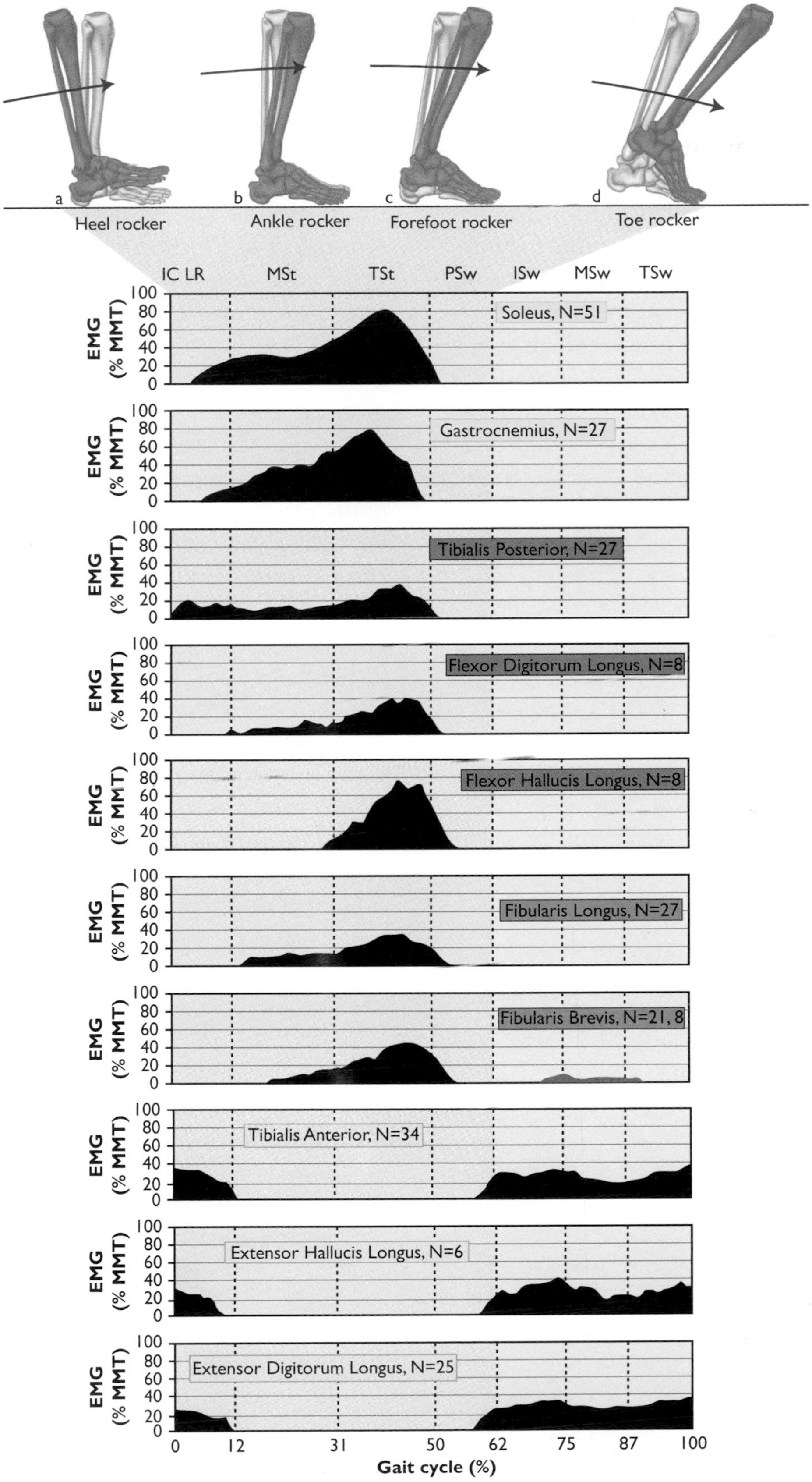

Figure 3.5. *From heel strike, the rest of the limb "vaults" over the rocker of the calcaneus (A) and progresses into dorsiflexion via the talar joint, which tensions the plantar flexors (B). As its natural range is met, the heel lifts to force the point of contact with the ground onto the rocker of the ball of the foot (C) and eventually onto the toes (D). (Adapted from Perry and Burnfield 2010.)*

compensate and create extra positive work (such as that needed to walk uphill), or they may need to control extra negative work (i.e., they concentrically or eccentrically contract to control and decelerate the momentum).

Muscle fibers may concentrically contract to accelerate or decelerate momentum, but the force of that contraction is transmitted through its associated tendon. The stiffness of each tendon is influenced by a range of factors, including length and thickness. A short, thick tendon will be stiffer than a long, thin one, and the muscle must control the appropriate strain in relation to momentum and desired range of motion. It is therefore possible that the muscle fibers concentrically contract as the overall tissue lengthens.

Whether the muscles lengthen, shorten, or remain isometric (in our case, we prefer isometric to maintain efficiency), the soleus, gastrocnemius, and fibularis longus all increase their tone with the progression into ankle dorsiflexion at mid-stance (12%; see fig. 3.4). As the ankle rocker action lengthens the soleus and gastrocnemius (see fig. 3.6), the foot will return to a neutral position by supinating

and reengaging the midtarsal joints. Ankle dorsiflexion will allow the continuity of the soleus, gastrocnemius, and plantar fascia to further support the many joints of the foot in order to give a smooth transition through the forefoot and toe rockers. If the mid-foot does not revert properly (i.e., if the midtarsal joints do not reengage into a locked position), undue stress may be placed on the plantar fascia, as it will be forced to become a main stabilizer of the foot.

Because the soleus, the deeper of the two calf muscles, attaches medially on the calcaneus, it also assists in drawing the heel bone out of eversion (see chapter 5 for a fuller breakdown of the reactions of the foot). The soleus will have the cooperation of the deep posterior compartment for this correction because of the angle at which the tendons of tibialis posterior and flexors hallucis and digitorum longus cross the subtalar joint. The deep posterior muscles also tension in sequence from heel strike (tibialis posterior—explored further below), through mid-stance (flexor digitorum longus), to late stance (flexor hallucis longus), as each of them has a role to play in the deceleration of dorsiflexion (12–31%) and eventually toe extension during late stance (31–62%).

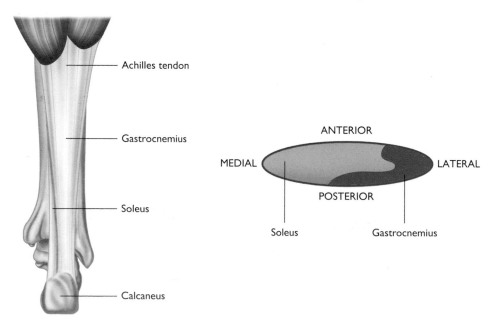

Figure 3.6. *Because of its deeper and more medial attachment, the soleus can help bring the calcaneus into inversion, thereby helping the tarsal bones to realign. The gastrocnemius attachments are more lateral and superficial, with much of its fascial tissue being continuous around the heel and into the plantar fascia (see fig. 3.8). (Adapted from Perry and Burnfield 2010.)*

Failure of any "rocker" will prevent the foot from rolling through onto the toes for an effective toe-off. The stride will naturally shorten, and often a hip-hiking strategy, whereby the affected limb is "lifted" from the same side of the pelvis through to flexion, will be used in compensation. This compensation may appear regardless of the cause (it could be due to a lack of hip extension, knee extension, or ankle dorsiflexion, or a loss of any of the foot rockers), and a strategy must therefore be developed for a differential diagnosis to create a remedial plan for the client.

Pulleys, the Windlass Effect, and Force Closure

As we saw in chapter 2, the foot experiences high forces following heel strike (0–2%) and in the build-up to toe-off (late stance 50–62%). The foot benefits from being relatively stable and supinated in both of these phases, but the mechanisms used to create stability at either end of stance are different. Prior to heel strike, there is tension in the tibialis anterior and extensors hallucis and digitorum longus to bring the foot into dorsiflexion and inversion during the swing phase (see fig. 3.4). The tension of these three muscles supports supination in preparation for heel strike.

However, the re-supination in preparation for toe-off is created through the tensioning of all the plantar flexors, as they control dorsiflexion and toe extension during the stance phase and the progression over the foot rockers.

Once the heel begins to rise during mid-stance, the foot should be stable to deal with the offset of forces (see fig. 2.28). As we progress onto the forefoot rocker, the point of support (the forefoot) is well in front of the body weight coming down to the ankle and a long lever is created. If the foot is unstable, it will struggle to transition through this phase and fail to distribute the resultant forces through the entire foot and ankle complex. The abilities to dorsiflex the ankle and extend the toes are essential events that create soft-tissue support and force closure of the foot to assist this mechanism (see fig. 3.7). Loss of range of motion in the foot rockers will have a detrimental effect on foot supination and stability.

The dorsiflexion of the ankle is symbiotic with the inversion of the bones of the feet; both events assist in tensioning the plantar tissue (see fig. 3.8). This gathering together of the bones of the foot and the tensioning of the elastic tissue create form closure to support the foot as a rigid lever.

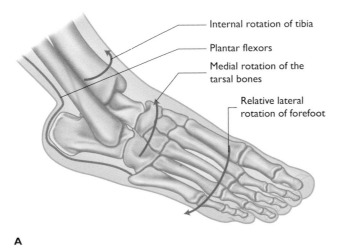

Internal rotation of tibia

Plantar flexors

Medial rotation of the tarsal bones

Relative lateral rotation of forefoot

A

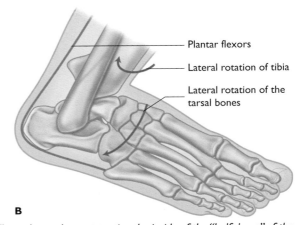

Plantar flexors

Lateral rotation of tibia

Lateral rotation of the tarsal bones

B

Figure 3.7. *The progression from plantar flexion to dorsiflexion (A to B) pulls on the tendons supporting the inside of the "half-dome" of the foot. All of the plantar flexors from each of the lateral, posterior, and deep posterior compartments will assist with drawing the bones of the pronated foot together to give it "force closure" and thereby assist with supination.*

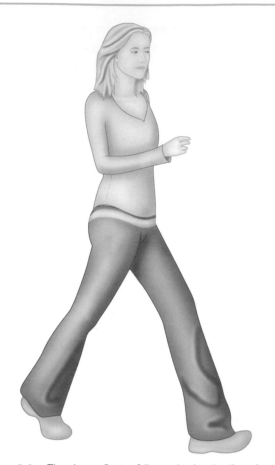

Figure 3.8. *The plantar flexion following heel strike (front foot) shortens the plantar flexors and allows the midtarsal joints and bones to open and adapt to the surface. Coming into dorsiflexion (back foot) tensions the soleus and gastrocnemius and thereby helps tension the plantar fascia, which draws the midtarsal bones back together and creates an integrated foot for toe-off, the so-called "windlass effect" (herein referred to as "force closure").*

The eponymous tendon may have been Achilles's weak spot but, thankfully for the rest of us, it is one of the strongest areas in our bodies. The fibers from the soleus and gastrocnemius spiral by approximately 90 degrees into the tendon (see fig. 3.6). This brings the soleus to the medial aspect of the calcaneus, where it can help produce inversion (Doral et al. 2010). Despite its great strength, however, the Achilles tendon is still the third most ruptured tendon in the body, after the rotator cuff and the tendons of the knee. This should not come as a surprise when we consider that it has to handle forces of up to twelve times our body weight, but, as we saw in chapter one (see fig. 1.26), the myofascial arrangement is such that it creates

a consistent increase in stiffness as it lengthens through its normal range.

The Achilles tendon, like the rest of the body, has been shown to be hugely adaptable, apparently increasing its cross-sectional area as usage increases. It has been found that the tendon in athletes is significantly thicker than in nonathletes. It should be noted, however, that the direction of correlation is not fully established; it could be that a thicker Achilles tendon leads to better athletic performance (Malvankar and Khan 2011). Studies have also shown that there is a feedback between the stiffness of the tendon and the tension of the attaching/controlling muscles and, as mentioned above, the muscles adjust their tension to match the elasticity of the tendon in order to maximize the efficiency of the elastic output (Lichtwark and Wilson 2007, Sawicki et al. 2009).

Force closure of the foot is reliant on the performance and strength of the Achilles tendon during toe-off. Progression through to the toe rocker will tension the tendon, reengage the midtarsal joints, and engage the plantar fascia. The lengthening created by the progressive dorsiflexion will load the tissue significantly, creating a tremendous amount of energy that can be utilized to push the body forward when it is released.

This makes the Achilles tendon, along with the gluteus maximus, one of the most important anatomical factors for human gait. The human Achilles tendon is much longer than that of other primates, and the calf is less bulky — much of the power is produced through elasticity rather than muscle contraction. This allows our lower leg to be lighter, which means that it takes less energy to move it. It also gives it the greatest velocity of any of our body parts, as well as the advantage of assistance from a larger tendon storage system. We see this dynamic to an even greater extent in the limbs of animals that use strong hip and thigh muscles to control their long, slender, and tendinous hind limbs, such as horses, antelopes, and kangaroos.

Catapults

The effect of the foot rockers and the tensioning of the tissue that occurs through ankle dorsiflexion and knee extension creates a catapult mechanism. The forward momentum of the tibia and femur is decelerated by the isometric contraction of the plantar flexors. This leads to the mechanical loading of the elastic tissues, which are stretched until being finally released at toe-off, once the foot has progressed over the toe rocker. The toes act as the final locking device, and once they are released, the stored energy in the elastic tissue assists with forward propulsion. This is triggered by full extension of the knee, which seems to allow the hamstring and gastrocnemius tissues to link together as a continuous system. Knee extension is necessary to properly load both the foot and ankle complex and the front of the hip; thus, in gait, knee extension is another "essential event" linking the foot and the hip, and loss of range at one joint inhibits the tissue loading ability of the other two joints.

Exercise 3.2. **Much of the force closure of the foot is created within the lower leg, but one can feel the loss of power brought about by a lack of knee extension by just taking a few steps without fully straightening the legs. Compare this to your normal gait (if you do bring the knee into extension!), and feel how the engagement of the fascia across the knee joint greatly assists the power of the plantar flexion. Some of this may be explained by knee flexion shortening the gastrocnemius and therefore taking it out of the equation, but even a slight change in knee position causes more change in power than one would expect. This may be due to the interlocking effect of the fascia from the hamstrings (see Myers 2009), but is more likely due to the simultaneous decrease in range of motion in the toes and hips as the pelvis progresses over the toe rocker, losing the power of toe-off.**

The catapult of the foot is assisted by a similar contrivance in the tissue that crosses the front of the hip—as the pelvis comes forward into hip extension, it stretches the myofascia of the anterior hip. It can do this because of the "lock" or "trigger" created by the foot on the ground, which prevents the leg from coming forward too early. Once the foot progresses onto the toe rocker, the two catapults are released simultaneously—one for hip flexion and one for foot flexion. You may have felt the loss of this force in exercise 3.2 as the two catapults work in concert, requiring the motion at the involved joints to be in balance in order to load and then release the springs effectively.

The tissue springs require the "trigger" mechanism of the toe rockers to propel the leg forward into flexion with ease. Theoretically, without the release of the foot created from the toe rocker, the elastic tension created by the hip extension would encourage movement of the pelvis backward rather than movement of the leg forward.

Catapult mechanisms have been discussed widely in the movement of other animals, but only rarely in that of humans. We adopt similar strategies, albeit with less-dramatic effects, to the huge leaps of bush babies and the phenomenal shooting of curled lizard tongues. Being less specialized, our springs are of a more sedate nature but are nonetheless important contributors to the spring motions we gain from our elastic tissues in the reduction of calorie expenditure.

The force closure and catapult reactions depend on a number of events—foot rockers all performing appropriately, as well as knee and hip extension—to bring the fascial tissues into engagement to allow momentum to assist the movement. Our range of motion is therefore crucial for graceful walking. Many experiments have been done comparing the efficiency of upright versus quadrupedal gait using trained chimpanzees. The design of the experiments was flawed from the start, because the chimpanzees' joints have different ranges from ours and therefore do not allow the same levels of fascial engagement to occur.

Chimpanzees have a range of 45 degrees of dorsiflexion, which allows their feet to grasp the trunk of a tree as they climb; this range is far beyond the 20 degrees in humans. For the catapult or elastic mechanism to work, we have to engage the fascial tissues in a stretch; a chimpanzee would require a very long stride to create enough dorsiflexion to pull on their Achilles tendon. Paleoanthropologists use ankle joints as an indicator of upright gait: by looking at the shape of the distal tibia, they can infer the joint's range of motion and the angle of transfer of force. In upright, bipedal gait, the body weight passes almost straight through the joint. In most quadrupeds, by contrast, it passes through the joint at an angle, since they remain more dorsiflexed as they move.

The first hominin fossil that we see with ankle joints that indicate a bipedal stance is "Lucy," possibly the world's most famous human ancestor, found by Donald Johanson in Ethiopia in 1974. Named after the Beatles' hit "Lucy in the Sky with Diamonds," Lucy has been confirmed as an example of *Australopithecus afarensis* and dates from approximately 3.2 million years ago. She was quite short, at around 3 feet 7 inches, and her bones exhibit many features that show that Lucy walked consistently on two legs, including pelvic, femoral, and humeral changes (many other primates are only occasional bipeds). Lucy is the oldest fossil showing some of these changes in the leg bones. Many older fossils also show some signs of bipedalism, though their remains are not as complete as Lucy's, with few lower limb bones surviving in the fossil record so far.

Although Lucy did not give us much information on the changes in the lower leg, other fossils have provided significant details on the evolution of its form and function. As the lower leg has the greatest velocity of any of our body parts during walking and running, minimizing its weight has many benefits for energy conservation. Evolving longer,

stronger tendons that can be used for greater energy storage diminishes the need for heavy muscles in the calf; moreover, the force per volume of muscle is optimized because the muscles of the calf are pennate (see chapter 6 for more information on the benefits of pennate muscles). We see this arrangement frequently in the rest of the animal world, such as in horses, antelopes, and kangaroos, which use their strong hip and thigh muscles to control long, slender, and tendinous limbs (see fig. 3.9). However, *Homo sapiens* tend to have shorter tendons, as we walk on our heels and only use the full elastic potential of the calf during running, especially if we run on our mid- or forefoot. Most other mammals locomote on some portion of their forefoot, further increasing the number of bent joints in need of control by their much larger proximal muscles.

If you revisit exercise 3.2, you may notice that not extending the knee coincided with decreased hip extension. This "bent-knee, bent-hip" gait is characteristic of nonhuman primates, but their use of this type of gait is due to their inability to create a lumbar lordosis rather than to a lack of length in the tissue. Because they cannot achieve simultaneous joint extensions and fully engage the long multi-joint myofascial tissues when walking upright, they rely much more on muscle power, without accessing the catapult mechanisms like we do.

Within his "Anatomy Trains" model, Myers (2015) discusses the concept of "expresses" versus "locals". He describes "local" muscles as those that cross one joint, and "expresses" as those that cross two or more. We can use this concept to explore the catapult phenomenon. By allowing the hip and knee joints to extend and the ankle to dorsiflex, the "expresses" engage more fully across these areas, with longer portions of the myofascial tissues being put under stretch. Without the stretch, the tissue will have to actively contract to produce the required force for flexion.

The long-chain stretches involved in an unrestricted stride reduce the load on the

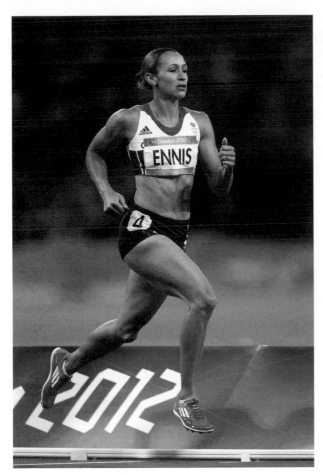

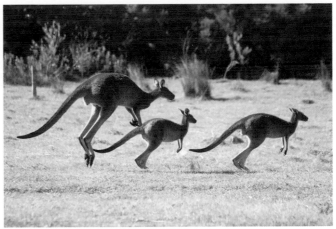

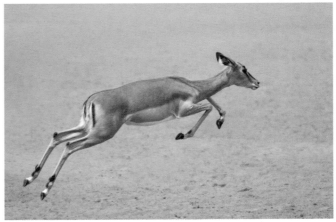

Figure 3.9. *As in all elite runners, in comparison to the bulk of her upper body, Jessica Ennis's lower leg appears quite spindly. When compared to the elite "athletes" of the nonhuman animal kingdom, this arrangement of proximal muscles controlling the long, tendinous sections of the lower leg seems common. (Jessica Ennis photograph courtesy of Getty Images. Kangaroo and antelope photographs courtesy of istock.com.)*

deeper, usually "local" muscles. In the absence of elastic energy, the muscles will have to work and thereby potentially become overused. As other primates cannot extend their knees and hips, their muscles are highly developed compared to ours.

It is important to remember, however, that the "engagement" might not be due to force transfer from one tissue to its neighbor. For example, the extension created through the body toward toe-off increases the stiffness in the anterior tissues and thereby enhances stability, such as when lumbar extension tensions the rectus abdominis, which pulls up on the pubis and counters the downward pull from the rectus femoris. If these two forces are in some form of balance, the pelvis will be able to communicate force between these two predominantly sagittal muscles. The same

argument can be made for many other areas of myofascial connection, and more research is needed to prove actual force transfer between myofascial units. The body does not require fascial continuity in order to increase stiffness—momentum and muscle contraction can provide it, but, if continuity is present, it is likely to enhance the potential catapult effect.

■ EVENTS AT THE IMPORTANT PHASES

Pre-Swing—Loading the Catapult to Release into Swing Phase

As the pelvis progresses over the foot, the knee begins to bend in the pre-swing phase, pushing out against the anterior fascia (see fig. 3.10). This further stimulates the connective tissue and could stimulate the muscles of the anterior compartment to contract in anticipation of lifting the foot and supporting it through the swing cycle. The extra fascial tension in the tibialis anterior may also have a role in the inversion/supination of the medial arch, bringing it out of the eversion/pronation pattern created following heel strike, though, as will be discussed later, it is more likely that there are stronger forces at work for that supination.

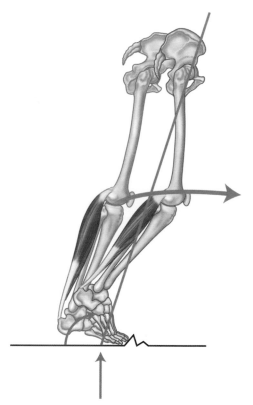

Figure 3.10. *When the knee comes forward to prepare for the leg swing, it will push into the anterior tissues (A), assisting with the lift of the leg and creating the signal for the muscles of the anterior compartment to begin contracting to lift and support the foot. EMG readings (see fig. 3.5) show the tibialis anterior and the long extensors all beginning to contract during the pre-swing phase and staying active until the weight is fully received by the foot in loading response. (After Perry and Burnfield 2010.)*

Heel Strike—Landing

Just as the anterior tissues assist the recoil for flexion, the posterior tissues help with extension. At heel strike, the foot is in front of the center of gravity and the hip is flexed, creating a lot of downward force behind

the body's point of contact with the ground (see fig. 3.11). There are a number of fascial arrangements that are automatically engaged in this position, the first of which might be the idea of the "Superficial Back Line" (SBL) but probably better combined with Vleeming's "Deep Longitudinal Sling" (DLS), which comprises the fibularis longus, biceps femoris, sacrotuberous ligament, and opposite erector spinae. With the hip flexed, the sacroiliac joint nutated, the knee extended, and the ankle dorsiflexed, the fascia of the SBL/DLS will be lengthened prior to heel strike. (As will be discussed later, many other tissues also make a strong contribution to resisting gravity's pull into hip flexion, and by decelerating hip flexion, they encourage the forward propulsion into hip extension.)

After being strongly loaded during heel strike, the extensor tissues now have to lengthen in

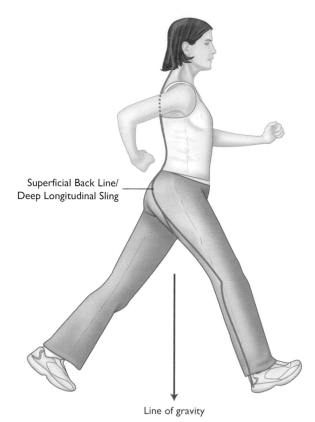

Superficial Back Line/ Deep Longitudinal Sling

Line of gravity

Figure 3.11. *In the position shown, the fascia of the Superficial Back Line/Deep Longitudinal Sling is tensioned by the flexion at the hip and ankle. This appears to stimulate the supporting muscles of the hamstrings from mid-swing through to loading response, when the body is much more aligned over the foot.*

the lower section, below the knee, as the ankle moves into dorsiflexion. Ankle dorsiflexion will lengthen all of the plantar flexors, including the fibulares, the tibialis posterior, and the flexors hallucis and digitorum longus. As these muscles come forward to their natural end of range, they will decelerate the tibia, while the femur progresses more quickly above, bringing the knee and hip joints into extension and simultaneously force closing the foot.

Swing Phase—Two Offset Forces

The pelvis moves in each dimension during gait: it has an overall anterior tilt in the sagittal plane, it tilts laterally (we explore this in the next chapter), and it rotates left to right. Strangely, much of the rotation introduced to the body in walking, particularly to the pelvis, is initiated by the sagittal plane elements of the flexors and extensors. The forward swing of one leg will pull the hip on that side forward, via the hamstring attachment, and the opposite side will be held back by the tensioning of the flexors as the hip goes into extension. The combined effect is therefore to rotate the pelvis, provided the stride is long enough to engage both lines of tissue. The contralateral forces of the opposing flexors and extensors are therefore essential for the creation of a series of events for the rest of the body, as they promote pelvic rotation to engage the body's many obliquely arranged fibers in the transverse plane (which we will explore in chapter 5).

When walking is observed from the side, there is an apparent 20-degree extension of the hip prior to toe-off. This is not pure extension, however, but rather an accumulation of events at different joints: the hip itself (which can extend by up to 10 to 12 degrees), the anterior tilt of the connecting ilium (between 3 and 7 degrees), and the backward rotation of the whole pelvis (between 8 and 12 degrees). The hip extension and the anterior tilt of the ilium serve to assist with the preloading of the superficial and deep flexors and oblique muscles (see chapters 5 and 6).

Rotation of the pelvis is required to help lengthen the stride: the pivoting action on the weight-bearing hip joint allows the opposite leg to reach further forward. Experiment by walking with and without left-to-right pelvic rotation to feel the difference; to progress forward in the sagittal plane, the pelvis assists by rotating in the transverse plane.

Stride length, provided it is long enough, creates rotation of the pelvis (see fig. 3.12). Rotation of the pelvis rotates the sacrum, and the transverse motion is transferred into the spine. As mentioned earlier, we walk to take our heads and hands to other places. For our eyes to focus on our goals, our heads have to remain relatively steady, and so this rotation in the body has to be reduced before reaching the head.

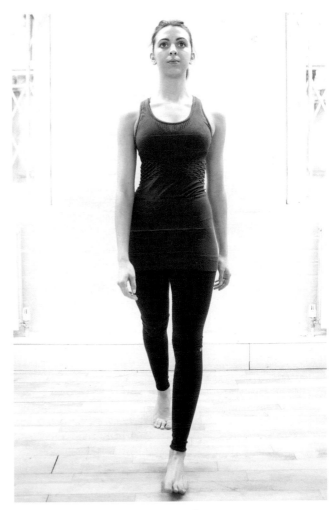

Figure 3.12. *Our bipedal gait naturally causes us to rotate as we reach forward with alternate legs. This rotation at the pelvis is useful for the transfer of force into the frontal and transverse plane tissues, but it must be reduced before reaching the head.*

During the swing of the leg forward toward heel strike, the posterior fascia on that leg is tensioned, which will contribute to the leg's ability to resist gravity once the calcaneus contacts the ground. Essentially, the flexion of the hip creates a pre-stretch of the hamstrings (as well as the other hip extensors) prior to heel strike. This serves to preload the fascial tissue and to enhance the power output of the antigravity muscles (the hamstrings, in this case), reducing the force they have to produce to prevent us falling to the ground.

The offset of deceleration forces during the swing phase also torsions the pelvis. As one leg swings through into hip flexion, the hamstrings will pull the ischial tuberosity with them, thereby encouraging the associated ilium into a posterior tilt. On the other side, the hip will be going into extension, so the hip flexors will be tautening and pulling their ilium into a relative anterior tilt.[5] The alternating and contralateral actions of the ilia create torsion within the pelvis, a movement that is allowed by the design of the sacroiliac joints at the back and the symphysis pubis at the front (see fig. 3.13).

Exercise 3.3. **Place your hands on your iliac crests and walk. Can you feel the movement of the ilia under the tissue? Do you sense the ilia tilting back as you swing the leg forward and then tilting forward as the thigh extends? The flexors and extensors therefore seem to be involved in creating this torsion action through the pelvis (see fig. 3.12, and explored further in the following chapters).**

The anterior tilt of the pelvis on the extended leg will tension—and thereby switch on—the abdominals on the same side. The ability of the pelvis to move is therefore essential to the functioning of the abdominals (and we will see later that the rotation and lateral tilt are necessary for the three dimensions of the

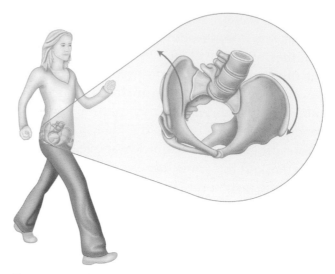

Figure 3.13. *Bipedal gait puts many vectors of force through the pelvis, requiring it to adapt in all three planes of motion (sagittal, frontal, and transverse). The lengthening and shortening of the flexors and extensors on alternate sides creates tilting in the sagittal plane, which leads to torsion in the pelvis.*

"core" to be activated). The overall anterior tilt of the pelvis creates extension in the back and tensions anterior musculature to assist with hip flexion via the mechanical link of the pelvis (see fig. 3.14).

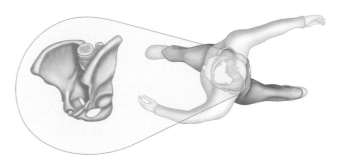

Figure 3.14. *While we walk, the pelvis is often in an overall anterior tilt (the posterior tilt of the ilium on the side of the flexed leg is relative to the resting tilt of the pelvis as a whole). As the leg extends, the pelvis acts as a mechanical link to connect the tensioning of the leg to the tissue of the torso, engaging the fascial elasticity.*

Exercise 3.4. **Place one hand on your abdominals and go for a short walk. Can you feel the tissue over the rectus abdominis becoming taut as either leg goes into extension? Experiment with different speeds—do you feel more or less fascial tensioning as you increase your speed?**

---

[5]We will revisit this in chapter 5—Transverse Plane—and discuss its significance for the sacroiliac joints.

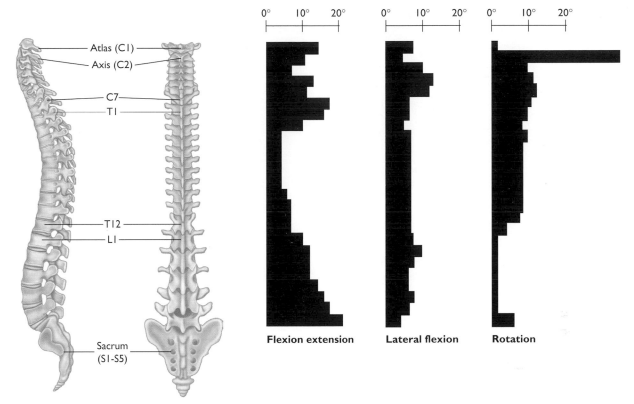

Figure 3.15. *Each spinal segment varies in its abilities to move in each plane. The lumbar spine does not have much rotation ability, so this will send the pelvic rotation up to the thoracic vertebrae. The increased amount of lumbar flexion and extension allows upright stance and long strides and also forms one of the 'essential events' for efficient gait.*

Although simplified,[6] fig. 3.15 shows the amount of rotation that is available at each spinal segment. Some of the rotation can be absorbed between L5/S1—the interface between the sacrum and the lowest lumbar vertebra—as it can rotate a few degrees, but the remaining rotational force will travel through the lumbars to reach the thoracics. The thoracic vertebrae have a much better range of motion in the transverse plane and are better able to reduce the rotation.

The facet joints of the lumbar vertebrae are predominantly arranged in the sagittal plane, allowing a wide range of flexion and extension—part of what allows us an upright, bipedal gait, as it gives us the ability to create lumbar lordosis (see fig. 3.16).

This arrangement restricts rotation, however, as the facets will encroach on one another in the transverse plane.

As we will see in chapter 5, the limitation of the lumbar spine is very useful: by encouraging the rotation up to the thoracics, it allows the contralateral forces of the oblique tissues to meet and recoil.

■ ESSENTIAL EVENTS

Toe-Off

At the point of toe-off, two catapult mechanisms have been created: one for toe-off and one for hip flexion—in the plantar flexors and hip flexors, respectively. The positional changes of the metatarsals we saw in chapter 2 are a vital component in the coupling between these two catapults, and, if we lose the ability to load one, we lose the efficiency of the other. Ideally, both of these catapult mechanisms are

---

[6]These data relate to the anatomical position and are therefore not entirely representative of the potential mechanics and range of motion of each joint when in motion. I have used them here to simplify the story and enhance understanding. For further information, please explore Gracovetsky's "Spinal Engine" (2008).

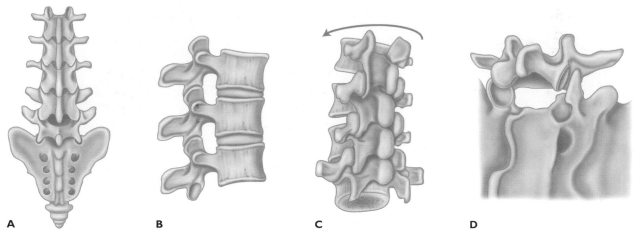

Figure 3.16. *The vertical orientation of most of the lumbar facet joints (A) allows a great deal of flexion and extension (B) but limits rotation, as they quickly interface with each other (C). The exception to this is the joint at L5/S1, which, because of L5's need to grab on to the tilted sacrum, has facets that are turned a little more to the frontal plane and can therefore allow a little more rotation between the two surfaces (D).*

discharged simultaneously, allowing the elastic energy of the calf and foot to produce plantar flexion and assisting the release of the hip flexors—each force encouraging the forward propulsion of the extended leg.

For that to happen, a number of sagittal plane events must take place. We need to roll through each of the foot rockers—heel, ankle, forefoot, and toe—and the knee and the hip must extend. The lumbar and thoracic spine must also extend. Finally, the head should preferably be kept upright to engage the anterior tissue and assist with flexion of the lower limb.

Heel Rocker

Our calcaneus is much larger than that of other primates, giving us a larger contact surface to dissipate the force at heel strike. This function is assisted by a thick pad of fat under the calcaneus (which absorbs approximately 17 to 19 percent of the impact force), and by the makeup of the bone itself, which is quite pliable. Any changes in either of these tissues, often as a result of localized trauma, can cause a protective limp to develop. The stride will shorten to avoid or minimize heel strike, and the contact time of the affected foot with the ground will decrease.

The rounded aspect of the calcaneus should be able to comfortably make contact with the ground and, because of its position behind the talar joint, encourage the foot to plantar flex and interface with the surface. Any number of factors may influence its ability to perform its duty as the first point of contact—heel spurs and plantar fasciitis being the two most common.

Ankle Rocker

Immediately following heel strike, the ankle should plantar flex by approximately 10 degrees, a movement controlled and decelerated by the anterior compartment (the tibialis anterior, in particular). Failure of these muscles leads to foot slap and the lack of proper absorption of the force of impact. Loss of function in these muscles is often due to neurological deficit (for example, a stroke or compartment syndrome–type compressions) and should therefore be managed by a physician.

The progression of the tibia and fibula over the talus can be restricted for a number of reasons. Apparent shortness in any of the tissues of the posterior and lateral compartments is the first and most obvious. Limits in these areas will also affect the transverse plane balance in the foot because of the medial and lateral pathways of the tissues around the ankle.

Since the talus is wider at the front of the bone than at the back, the tibial and fibular malleoli must spread in order to accommodate the talus in dorsiflexion (see fig. 3.17A). This mortise-and-tenon design means that when the foot is dorsiflexed, the talus is locked for extra ankle stability. The spreading of the malleoli requires both the adaptability of the interosseous membrane between the two bones and the ability of the fibula to move on the lateral aspect of the proximal tibia. While soft-tissue manipulation and stretching may be effective in dealing with limits in myofascial range, some form of bone manipulation may be required if the dorsiflexion is restricted by the joint interface. Dorsiflexion restriction can be due to congenital issues, if the talus is too wide or too flat at the front to interface correctly between the malleoli. In these cases, slight heel lifts may be a possible solution; these will provide relative dorsiflexion and reduce any compensation into pronation and medial toe-off.

The differences in causes of the limits can be assessed using a simple knee bend or squat, as described in fig. 3.17B.

The less common problem of too much dorsiflexion may lead to overuse strains on the posterior myofascia and is only an issue during high or increased usage.

Forefoot Rocker

Prior to toe-off, body weight should ideally progress onto the first and second metatarsal heads. The first metatarsal is wider and stronger than any of the other toes and is clearly designed to carry more force through it; however, in order to create a stable toe-off, its length needs to be relatively matched to that of the second metatarsal.

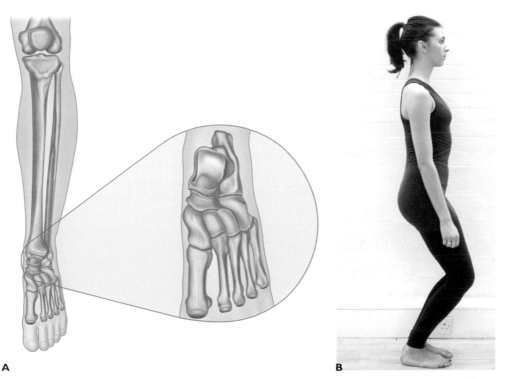

A **B**

Figure 3.17. *A, The tibia and fibula must be able to separate slightly on dorsiflexion to accommodate the greater width at the front of the talus. Limitations can develop within the interosseous membrane or at the proximal tibiofibular joint, but these can often be manipulated to improve range. Bony changes at the front of the talus may also occur, either acquired or present from birth, creating permanent restriction. B, When the client squats to the end of range in dorsiflexion, he or she may feel a "block" either behind the ankle (usually indicating a soft-tissue problem) or at the front (which is likely an indication of a joint restriction).*

In the 1920s, physician and evolutionary anatomist Dudley J. Morton discovered that approximately 15 percent of the population has what came to be known as *Morton's Foot*. In this condition, the second metatarsal is more than 8 millimeters longer than the first, and when the foot progresses toward toe-off, it will be doing so on a single point rather than two. This encourages the foot to "fall" to one side or the other, leading to a rotation (see fig. 3.18). If the metatarsals are of significantly different lengths, an orthotic correction (a Morton's extension) may be necessary.

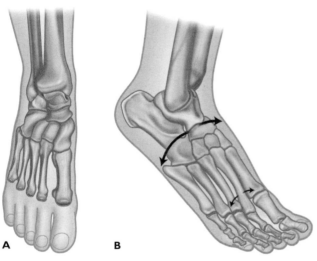

A   **B**

Figure 3.18.   Ideally, the first and second metatarsals will be of equal length (A), which will create a stable platform for toe-off. When the second metatarsal (or, less commonly, the first) is longer (B), an unstable, single point of contact is created prior to toe-off, encouraging the foot to progress more medially or laterally.

Imbalances can also be caused by changes in the soft tissue, especially with a high arch pattern and short plantar fascia. This functional (rather than structural) imbalance can often cause the toe-off to occur over the third, fourth, and fifth metatarsal heads rather than the first and second. This leads to a reduction in the amount of power produced in the myofascial trigger at toe-off, which may have to be compensated for by more work being produced elsewhere—often in the hip flexors.

Toe-off on the medial aspect of the big toe can lead to the development of hallux valgus (bunion), and, without sagittal plane progression over the first and second toes, torsion forces may be produced at the knee, causing a knee valgus pattern and thus creating issues for the ligaments (especially medial) and/or the menisci (lateral) (see fig. 3.19).

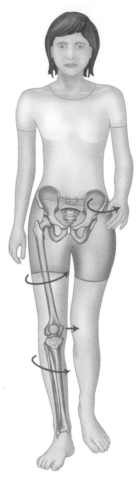

Figure 3.19.   Toeing off via the medial aspect of the big toe creates torsional forces for the first metatarsophalangeal joint (usually leading to hallux valgus) and a valgus force at the knee. This can lead to increased strain on the medial ligaments, because of the opening of the joint on the medial side, along with the possible compression of the lateral meniscus, because of the closing of the joint on that side.

This dynamic can be exaggerated by wearing shoes with pointed or restricted toe boxes. Crushing the phalanges can mechanically misalign the foot, leading to further joint distress with the added forces of walking. A wide toe box that allows the metatarsals to spread is ideal, not just for the joint alignment but also to stimulate the interossei, which have a reflex relationship with the quadriceps. As the metatarsals spread, mechanoreceptors in the tissue between them sense the movement and relay the impulse to the knee extensors to absorb the forces of gravity and ground reaction force (Michaud 2011).

Toe-off is most efficient if done on a platform of two metatarsal heads, and these will need to be in alignment in the sagittal and frontal planes. Unfortunately, another common metatarsal misalignment is a "plantar flexed first ray" (the ray being the line of bones of the first metatarsal and medial cuneiform). This is apparent when the head of the first metatarsal remains below the line of the others when the foot is held in neutral. The effect on the frontal plane rocker depends on whether the first ray is mobile, semiflexible, or fixed in plantar flexion. If the ray is fixed, it will force the foot to supinate and toe off laterally. If it is mobile, the foot will be more likely to roll medially and into pronation (possibly encouraging a hallux valgus). A semiflexible first ray is less traumatic for the rest of the foot biomechanics, but can lead to excess impact to the sesamoid bones if the first ray is unable to rise enough on impact as the foot rises through the toe rocker (see fig. 3.20).

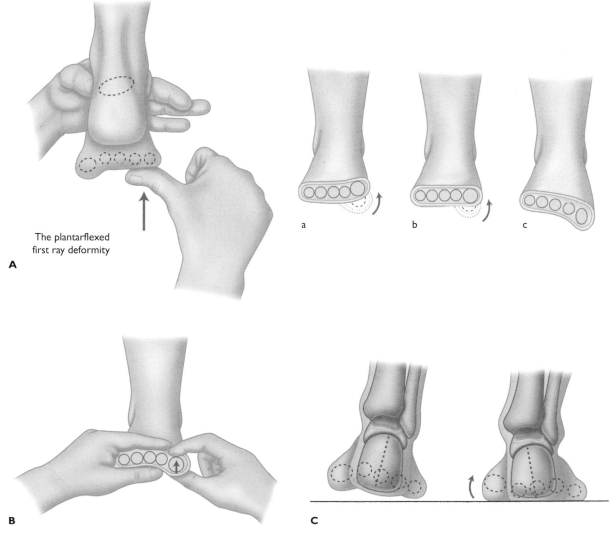

Figure 3.20. A, When the foot is aligned in neutral and the first ray remains below the level of the others, it should be checked for mobility (B), if it is hypermobile and rises above the level of the others (a–c), it can create instability of the first ray and lead to pronation. If it is fixed (C), the reverse will occur, and the foot will progress into supination as it is forced laterally. When the first metatarsal is only semimobile, coming into line with the others, impact forces will be transferred to the underlying sesamoids, creating inflammation that may lead to other compensations and limping. Resolution of these patterns may involve the fibularis longus muscle, as well as manipulation of the joints, if they are restricted. (Adapted from Michaud 2011.)

Toe Rocker

The first and second metatarsophalangeal joints must be in balance with one another and must be able to reach 40 to 55 degrees of extension. Any reduction in this range will lead to compensations, usually within the transverse plane. Also, recall that the rectus femoris is only switched on in the last few degrees of hip extension—a range dependent on toe extension (fig. 3.4). If we lose toe extension, the recruitment of the rectus femoris may be inhibited.

Hallux rigidus is a fusion at the first metatarsophalangeal joint with little possibility of correction and therefore requires adaptation of the environment—either changing to footwear that incorporates a toe-spring or using orthotics.

Hallux limitus simply refers to any reduction in extension ability of the big toe below the 40- to 45-degree ideal necessary for toe-off. The reasons for its development may be many, and a full orthopedic investigation may be required to check for bony changes. Manipulative intervention can include treatment of any and all of the big toe flexors, especially the flexor hallucis brevis.

Knee Extension

As the leg swings through before heel strike, the knee will gradually come into extension. We will revisit this in later chapters, where we will see that knee extension allows potential communication between the biceps femoris and the fibularis muscles, and between the adductor magnus and the deep posterior compartment. Knee extension may also be a useful addition to help distribute some of the contraction force from the hamstrings. The hamstrings' interlocking with the tissue of the gastrocnemius at the moment of heel strike allows the calf tissue to help stabilize the limb and absorb some of the force. As a bonus, it might help initiate knee flexion, along with the force of gravity.

Immediately after heel strike, the knee will flex by approximately 20 to 25 degrees to absorb the associated forces, and then gradually straighten again prior to heel lift. As discussed above, the flexion will assist with the extension through the recoil of elastic energy, and then, once the leg is straight, other body segments can communicate force across the knee and allow the knee extensors to be relatively passive.

Prior to heel lift, the knee flexes and the foot plantar flexes simultaneously, and it appears that we use the gastrocnemius to control both of these events: the power will be assisted by many other myofascial elements, but the coordination between these two events is strongly influenced by the "express" of the calf muscle. Factors that limit the extension of the knee could include lack of range in the gastrocnemius, chronic contracture of the hamstrings, and joint dysfunctions involving the menisci, cartilage, or ligaments. These deficiencies can be tested by using a range of loaded and unloaded assessments to differentiate the tissues that may be involved.

Research has shown that walking with a knee-bent gait leads to an increased usage of oxygen by up to 50 percent, illustrating the extent of the inefficiency of this type of gait, compared to allowing the knee to fully extend (Michaud 2011). This is further evidenced by the differences in strength between the other primates and humans. The average chimpanzee is much stronger than the average human; this is a result of a combination of genetic variance and muscle architecture. While chimpanzees also have pennate muscles—muscles with fibers aligned at an angle to the line of pull, which increases muscle efficiency—their fibers tend to be longer, allowing them to produce more power over a greater range. Chimpanzees also have higher levels of a gene called *ACTN3*, which creates more muscular muscles. In humans, ACTN3 is found in higher levels in sprinters and much lower levels in endurance runners; therefore, the level may be related to the fascial/muscle fiber balance within the soft tissues (Hawks 2009). The greater muscular strength of chimpanzees and other apes allows them to be comfortable walking with bent knees and hips.

Hip Extension/Flexion

Extension at the hip joint is restricted to approximately 10 degrees because of the strong iliofemoral ligament, so to increase the length of a step, we combine hip extension with a blend of pelvic tilt and rotation (see fig. 3.21). When extending the hip, we engage the iliofemoral ligament and the rectus femoris, and we draw on the fascia of the torso, meaning that the tissue of the rectus abdominis helps with hip flexion (see exercise 3.4). Any limitations in hip extension will limit the recoil into hip flexion and reduce the available momentum for the swing period.

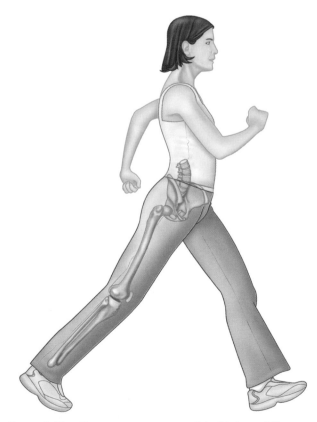

Figure 3.21. *The apparent extension of the hip is partially created by the pelvis tilting and rotating. Limitations in hip extension will often force the pelvis to tilt or rotate further, probably increasing the stresses on the lumbar and thoracic spines. A limitation in hip extension can also lead to a shorter stride, which may fail to rotate and torsion the pelvis, reducing the elastic loading of the other myofascial lines in the upper body and thereby increasing the work being done by the leg (including the psoas).*

Similarly, a lack of hip flexion will limit the amount of pre-tensioning placed on the extensors. A lack of hip flexion will also reduce the length of the lever created at heel strike, as the foot will be placed closer to the body's center of gravity, and will therefore require less work to be done to resist gravity and produce hip extension. This will force the posterior chain muscles to work harder, and the gait will look labored, compared to the ease of someone fully engaging their fascial spring mechanisms.

The use of the springs of the flexors and extensors allows minimal contractions in hip and knee muscles, and, if orchestrated correctly, the foot progresses with just 1.29 centimeters of ground clearance (Michaud 2011). The range of each of the lower limb flexions is kept small and not consciously created, but produced instead by the release of the "trigger" of the toe rocker. One quickly feels the difference between walking on a smooth surface and walking on an uneven surface that requires greater ground clearance and therefore more muscle effort.

Lumbar Extension

As discussed above, lumbar extension is one of the unique human traits that permits bipedal gait, since it enables us to stand upright and also allows the pelvis to tilt anteriorly as we step forward. If the lumbars are extended because of an anteriorly tilted pelvis or a posteriorly tilted rib cage, they may limit the amount one is able to extend his or her hip and draw on the front of the pelvis (see fig. 3.22).

Thoracic Extension and Head Position

Exercise 3.1 demonstrated the relationship of head and trunk position to the power of hip flexion or its connection to it. An anterior head position and/or limited extension in the

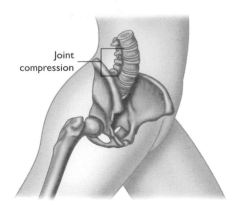

Joint compression

Figure 3.22. An anteriorly titled pelvis leads to further lumbar extension, which may reduce the amount of available hip extension if the hip flexors are shorter than normal. The relative range of motion may also adjust to produce the appearance of greater range in extension and a limitation in flexion. The therapist's attention should first be on repositioning the pelvis rather than on hip flexor/extensor balance, provided that resting lengths are within normal limits.

thoracic spine should be addressed to reduce strain in the deep hip flexors. If the flexors cannot fully and properly engage, hip flexion may be initiated through muscular effort instead of through fascial recoil, which would lead to overuse.

An anterior head position and/or limited thoracic extension may be produced by anything that draws the head down and compresses the front of the rib cage, in which case any superficial tissue may engage quite early in hip extension. If the client is unable to fully extend the hip, the flexors may not be correctly loaded and will be less economical in their assistance with hip flexion. This scenario could lead to an overuse of the flexors or to a rotational strategy, in which the client turns the limb (internally or externally) to avoid the limitations in flexion or extension. Rotational compensation can be used to work around a lack of any of the sagittal plane events, especially at the foot and the hip. When medial or lateral deviations are noticed (particularly when they are more apparent functionally compared to structurally), each of the sagittal plane "essential events" should be assessed for range and quality of motion.

■ SUMMARY

1. In-series joint alignment determines overall movement direction—crabs cannot walk straight ahead, as their joints are aligned laterally.
2. Each of the sagittal plane "essential events" is necessary for the full involvement of the flexors and extensors, allowing them to utilize the full potential energy created through myofascial pre-tensioning or strain.
3. In developing an upright, bipedal gait, our alignment with gravity became more centralized than that of the primate knuckle walkers and arboreal quadrupeds. Although our evolution of bipedal gait has removed some degree of stability, it has allowed us the ability to use forward movement to load fascial continuities with elastic energy. It is as if our skeleton strains (in a good way!) the fascial tissues by walking into them, the pelvis pushing back or forward to create length and the muscles adjusting the tension to minimize the work involved in keeping us upright and moving forward.
4. Gravity loads the tissue in response to the resistance of ground reaction forces, and the propulsion forward or backward creates slings to catapult us forward. These elastic, myofascial catapults are controlled by certain triggers, the greatest one being toe-off, which releases the energy simultaneously from the hip flexors and the plantar flexors.
5. The essential events that allow us to take advantage of sagittal plane efficiency mechanisms are: each of the foot rockers (heel, ankle, forefoot and toe), knee extension, hip extension and spinal extension (especially lumbar).

As we will see in chapters 4 and 5, the pelvic and hip joints also create elastic loading for myofascial tissue in the frontal and transverse planes, and, once we have these in balance, we will have a full understanding of the "spring in our step."

4

FRONTAL PLANE

It's Niagara Falls. It's one of the most beautiful natural wonders in the world. Who wouldn't want to walk across it?

—Nik Wallenda

▪ INTRODUCTION

While the sagittal plane was about momentum, the frontal plane is about the balancing act necessitated by the offset between ground reaction force coming up to the hip joint and our center of gravity somewhere in our lower abdomen. While few of us want to walk across Niagara Falls on a tightrope, we all have a range of skeletal characteristics that allow our feet to land relatively close to the midline. Having our center of support below our center of gravity makes functional sense, and it comes with the added benefit of pre-tensioning many of the muscles involved in supporting us through the single-leg stance period of gait.

The abductors on the stance side are pre-tensioned by a side-to-side tilt of the pelvis, which is one of the main frontal plane events during gait. This side-to-side action—provided it can be controlled to around 4 degrees of tilt—supplies extra tissue stiffness to the abductors

as they assist the control of the pronation cascade. There are a few essential events without which the side-to-side tilt of the pelvis will be inhibited. These include:

- Side flexion of the lumbar spine
- Hip adduction of the stance limb
- Hip abduction of the opposite limb

▪ MOVEMENT AIDS ECONOMY

In chapter three we explored the benefits of in-series pre-tensioning of tissues oriented to the sagittal plane, and saw how the sagittal tissues benefit from loading in response to forward momentum. The frontal plane tissues use more of the counterpoise between ground reaction force coming up from the lower limb and the body's mass coming down from its center of gravity and how the offset causes the pelvis to tilt. While sometimes considered a negative feature, we will see how the tilt actually initiates efficiency mechanisms for the body.

With each step, we have to stop ourselves from falling. When the foot hits the ground, a significant downward force is absorbed by the body's soft tissues, and while much of that work is sagittal and performed by the hip and knee extensors, the hip abductors are required to prevent adduction in the frontal plane. As we saw in chapter 1, it is this folding of the joints—an inherent instability in the system—that provides shock absorption (i.e., it protects the brain from jiggling around) and also provides metabolically cheap elastic energy. The downward motion loads the springs within the myofascia (see fig. 4.1), and so the "falls" are not a bad thing—they are caused by offsets of force across joints, and they provide myofascial efficiency.

As the swing leg progresses past the rockers of the planted foot, a gentle rise of the body is created as the body comes over the forefoot of the planted foot. The body lowers again at heel strike. This upward and downward movement appears to assist much of the loading of the elastic tissues to take advantage of the stretch-shortening cycle. The rise of the body is necessary to create the potential energy that turns to kinetic (i.e., moving) energy on the fall, and the deceleration of this momentum is what feeds the stretch of the elastic tissues to provide the elastic recoil.

A study by Ortega and Farley (2005) showed that reducing vertical displacement of the head (i.e., the up/down "bounce" of walking) increased the metabolic cost of walking—the muscles had to work harder. Increased energy use with less vertical movement seems contradictory to traditional thinking, which would suggest minimizing up/down movement would be more energy efficient. However, just as momentum is needed by the body to create the pre-stretch in the elastic tissue in the sagittal plane, vertical oscillation also plays a role in our bipedal efficiency. The oscillation generated by the interaction of gravity and ground reaction force provides momentum to create pre-tensioning of the tissues in the same manner as the body's forward movement.

Vertical displacement is related to body size and speed: if we increase speed, we also increase vertical movement, giving us more

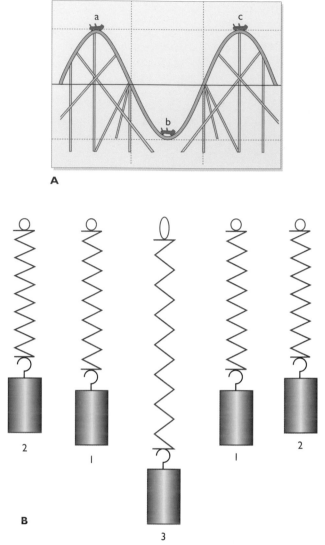

Figure 4.1. *A, As the roller-coaster car glides down the track (from a to b) it builds the kinetic energy used to ascend the next rise (to c). At the top, much of the kinetic energy has been used up (as work), but, because of its new position on the apex of the ride, the car now has a lot of potential energy. This potential energy quickly becomes kinetic energy, once the car is on the downward side of the rise and starts to accelerate. B, The downward motion of the weight is decelerated by the resistance of the spring. The kinetic energy of the downward movement transfers into the spring, which reaches a point at which the force applied by the weight is matched by the elastic strength of the spring. Once the two forces are matched no more downward movement occurs. The lowest point of the bounce of the spring is the same point as the roller coaster being at the top of the rise—we now have enough potential energy stored in the spring to "bounce" the weight back up.*

downward momentum to stretch and load the elastic tissues to provide kinetic energy on their release. This change in strategy may explain some alterations we see in gait as speed increases. Increased efficiency following locomotor gear change was noticed by Hoyt and Taylor (1981), who measured the energy costs of different speeds for ponies. They found that the animals chose the particular speed for each pattern of gait—walk, trot, or gallop—that was the most energy efficient: the different styles of movement led to optimum elastic loading (see fig. 4.2).

Hoyt and Taylor (1981) found that the ponies' energy costs increased with an increase in speed for each style of gait; furthermore, when the gait pattern changed from a walk to a trot and from a trot to a gallop, there was a decrease in metabolic cost (fig. 4.2A). Each transition reduced the amount of effort: a slow trot required less effort than a fast walk, and a slow gallop was also metabolically cheaper than a fast trot. When these data are analyzed for the variation in cost relative to distance (fig. 4.2B), we see that each gait pattern uses the same ratio of energy to distance (approximately 300 joules per meter). It is also interesting to note that walking has a very narrow range of efficiency (shown by the length of the bar at the bottom of the graph in fig. 4.2B) compared to trotting and galloping. The efficiency of walking for horses is very sensitive to changes in speed.

You can feel this dynamic yourself by going for a walk and gradually speeding up. When you are going fast enough, you will naturally switch to a jog, then to a run, and eventually to a sprint. After each change, you can feel that you regain some efficiency, as the progression allows you to take advantage of the stretch-shortening cycle, reducing muscle effort. It is important to remember, however, that factors other than speed will be involved in this, including muscle strength and biomechanics. This book predominantly traces the most efficient and common biomechanical paths that take advantage of the myofascial tissues.

■ GETTING STARTED—2—WITH GRAVITY

The longest journey begins with a single step.

—Lao Tsu

Before we change speed, we must first start walking; we saw the benefits of sagittal preloading for the initiation of gait in chapter 3, but we also gain from preloading in the frontal plane. A lateral transfer of body weight onto our swing leg before we begin walking creates vertical loading of the limb and tensions the lateral tissues, by creating a slight adduction on the weight-bearing hip.

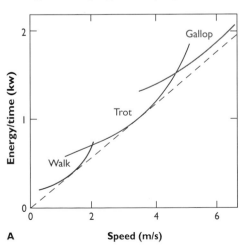

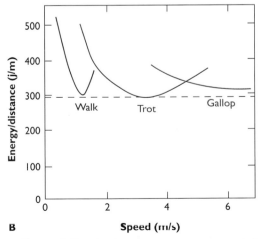

A

B

Figure 4.2. *A, Energy costs as a function of speed for three gait patterns of horses. B, Variation in energy costs per meter relative to speed for horses. (Adapted from Hoyt and Taylor 1981.)*

When standing and intending to take a step, our body weight shifts briefly (and unconsciously) from being centrally placed between the feet toward the leg to be lifted, before transferring across to the weight-bearing side (see fig. 4.3). The weight shift prior to initiation suggests that vertically loading the swing leg may assist with recoiling it up and forward while simultaneously loading the myofascia of the lower limb.

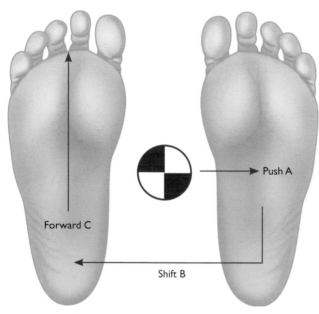

Figure 4.3.   *Pressure plate analysis shows that, in preparation for the first step, we move our center of gravity onto the swing leg momentarily before bringing it onto the stance side to initiate the step. This may help to mechanically load the tissue of the swing leg to assist with lifting and propelling it forward. By bringing the body weight onto the swing leg, the tissues will be loaded and potentially deformed a little to provide a spring to assist its first lift. (Adapted from Perry and Burnfield 2010.)*

■ IT'S ALL IN YOUR HEAD

Brain size is often used as a species indicator by scientists studying the ancestral hominid lineage. Along with other morphological indicators, brain size has been used to differentiate the *Homo* genus from the earlier *Australopithecus*—and from *Ardipithecus* before them (see fig. 4.4). Few people realize, however, that our extinct cousins, the Neanderthals—with whom we shared the world for around three hundred thousand years—not only had

larger, more muscular bodies than *Homo sapiens* but also had larger brains. Why, then, were we able to outlast our brainier and brawnier cohabitants?

In *Anatomy Trains*, Myers (2015) describes how the multipurpose sensory organs of the ear lie along our lateral aspects, and this could be where we had our competitive advantage. As Myers (2015) and McCredie (2007) point out, the sides of our bodies have their evolutionary origin in the lateral lines of fish, in which organs are embedded that perceive vibrations from the surrounding environment. These piscine sensory organs evolved into the human ear, with its ability not only to hear but also to sense orientation and movement. The semicircular canals (SSCs) are an important part of this system and lie within the inner ear and cooperate with the eyes and sub-occipital muscles to create the vestibulo-ocular reflex to stabilize vision during eye and head movement.

The SCCs are an essential part of the vestibular system for balance and orientation (fig. 4.5). As part of the inner ear, the three fluid-filled canals are oriented to the sagittal, frontal, and transverse planes, with each movement plane officially termed *pitch*, *roll*, and *yaw* in relation to their function. When movement occurs in one of the planes, it causes the canal to move further than the endolymph fluid that is contained within and creates relative motion between the two. The relative movement stimulates stereocilia within the ampulla, which then signal the brain regarding direction and amount of movement.

Fred Spoor, now of the Natural History Museum, London, has done much work investigating the role of the SCCs, with comparative studies between different species and their movement styles. Spoor (2003) found that, although the actual size of the SCCs increases with body size as one might expect, the relationship between the SCC size and body size was not always in the same ratio.

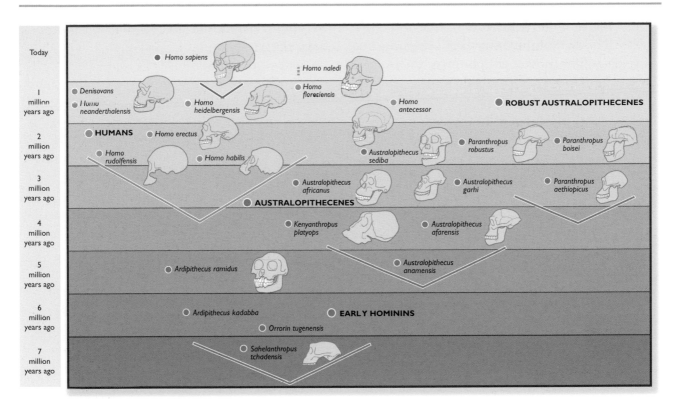

Figure 4.4. A hypothetical hominin family tree.

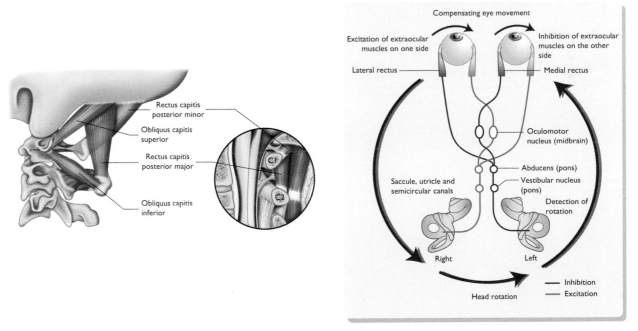

Figure 4.5. The vestibular system and the vestibulo-ocular reflex.

When plotting variations in movement styles of 91 primates (fast to extra slow; see fig. 4.6*A*) relative to body mass and SCC radius, there was an obvious best fit trend, with the more agile species having relatively larger than expected SCCs. An obvious comparison can be made between the bush baby (*Galago*), a fast and agile jumper, and the slow loris (*Nycticebus*), a particularly slow and ponderous mover (which, unfortunately, makes it popular with some dubious pet owners) (fig. 4.6*B*). These two animals have similar body mass but very dissimilar movement patterns: the *Galago* uses a fast and powerful elastic jumping action to catch its insect prey, in marked contrast to the laborious progress of the *Nycticebus*. One reason for their differing strategies may lie in their body mass/SSC ratio.

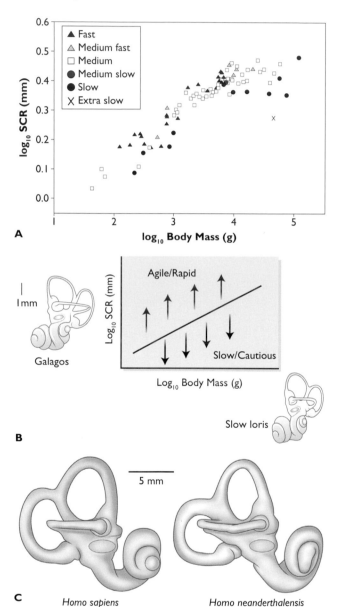

A

B

C   Homo sapiens   Homo neanderthalensis

Figure 4.6. *A, Chart showing the distribution of primate body mass (g) with respect to SCC radius (mm) to log10, and plotted according to locomotor type. B, The best fit line for 4.6A shows a trend that agile and rapid movement correlates with relatively larger SCC, as demonstrated by the bush baby and slow loris. C, Homo sapiens and Homo neanderthalensis show a similar disparity in the radius of SCC except for the lateral arc (responsible for sensing transverse plane movement), which is larger in Neanderthals (Spoor et al. 2003).*

Recent investigations on Neanderthal skulls have shown that their SCCs were smaller and less developed than those of *Homo sapiens* (fig. 4.6*C*). Balance, coordination, running, and throwing would presumably have been more difficult for them (although not impossible). An analysis of Neanderthal skeletons shows a similar kind of wear and tear, injuries, and arthroses to that experienced by today's rodeo riders, presumably caused by the need to get close enough to their prey to jab them with spears (McCredie 2007; Wynn and Coolidge 2012).

Compare that to the picture of *Homo sapiens* painted by Bramble and Lieberman (2004) and by McDougall (2010) of a graceful and elegant distance runner bounding from boulder to boulder and hurdling tree roots. Persistence hunting involves chasing prey to exhaustion and death, and, when coupled with the need for accurate throwing of spears and shooting of arrows, it is obvious that hunter-gatherers require a high level of balance and coordination. It has been proposed that humans' superior inner-ear apparatus gave us all of these abilities, along with enhanced navigational skills. The ability to find our way back to camp after chasing an antelope for many miles would be a welcome addition to the toolbox of any persistence hunter, and a larger inner ear certainly enables this. In contrast, the evidence of Neanderthal lifestyle seems to show that they rarely traveled far from their main encampment (Wynn and Coolidge 2012).

Furthermore, having a better developed proprioceptive sense (the perception of where one's body is in space) allows our brains to carry on with other jobs, as we no longer have to pay as much conscious attention to the surrounding environment and our relationship to it. This is exemplified by the case of Ian Waterman, a man whose brain lost the ability to receive many of the nerve signals from his body—while not paralyzed, he could not feel his body's existence and could not instinctively move it. Mr. Waterman was able to teach himself how to walk again, but walking required his full concentration and reliance on visual input; when distracted, he would fall, and trying to move in the dark would be impossible (Muller and Schleip 2011).

Perhaps *Homo sapiens* was able to find an effective (I hesitate to say "ideal") balance between brain and brawn by developing proprioceptive and coordinating abilities. Evolution and function are difficult to tie down to just a handful of factors, as many serendipitous and contingent evolutionary events were required for our ability to walk, talk, and throw all at the same time. However, the increase in the functional ability of our inner-ear system must have contributed significantly. It allowed us to take advantage of our elastic tissue, since moving elastically requires more deviation from the midline and allows us to use the momentum of our bodies in different ways, as in gymnastics or parkour. Furthermore, the less we have to think about moving, the better we will be at the many other requirements of life, adding to our efficiency. Having less brain processing tied up with spatial awareness is likely to have given us more adaptability.

It is estimated that the average calorie intake of Neanderthals, with their heavy, muscular builds and large bones, would have been between 3,500 and 5,500 calories per day, mostly gained from a variety of meat sources (Wynn and Coolidge 2012). It is easy to extrapolate that our lighter and more elastic frames required a lower daily calorie intake (2,000 to 3,000), while our greater spatial awareness gifted us with both a wider range of motion and the ability to maintain larger territorial maps in our minds. In essence, the combination of our inner-ear advances and our lighter frames gave us definite evolutionary advantages.

So, why is *Homo sapiens* the only extant hominin species? We have explored a few factors that may be involved, and, if we look back at fig. 4.4, we see significant developments in skull shape and changes in the proportions between the skull and the cranium. Starting at the very bottom of the chart with *Sahelathropus tchadensis* (an early biped but not necessarily an ancestor of our species), we see a very small, shallow brain case. As we progress up to the right with "Robust Australopithecines", there is a slight expansion of the brain case and therefore cranial capacity, along with a significant increase in the size of the jaw. The *Homo sapiens* group directly above *S. tchadensis* all have an expanded brain case and a reduced jaw. It is therefore tempting to conjecture a chain of adaptations which led to a more gracile human form that was both more efficient and more agile than our robust cousins, with increased brain capacity and larger SSCs. The symbiotic adaptations of increased brain capacity, SSC ratio, elasticity, and endurance running paint a convincing picture of an evolution toward more efficient and dynamic movement capabilities driven by myofascial mechanisms. However, as tempting as that story may be, it is impossible to know for sure.

■ PELVIC STABILITY

It don't mean a thing (if it ain't got that swing).

—Duke Ellington and Irving Mills

The adaptation of the inner ear is not the only lateral feature to contribute to our bipedal success. As we saw earlier, standing on one leg requires the ilia to face laterally to provide frontal plane stability. The femur's inward angle from the hip to the knee allows us to align our feet more directly under our center of gravity (see fig. 4.7), but the alignment also requires more work to resist gravity.

When we walk, the position of our feet moves inward, closer to our center of gravity compared to our "anatomical neutral" (i.e., standing upright), and we shift our body weight laterally with each step to better align our center of gravity above our center of support. The lateral shift of the pelvis pushes the greater trochanter out against the band of tissue of the abductors, whose most obvious role in walking is in supporting the pelvis in the frontal plane. The deltoid of the hip abductors—tensor fasciae latae (TFL), gluteus medius, and gluteus maximus—is called into play, preventing the pelvis from dropping too far into adduction at heel strike and into the swing phase, when the body weight is carried on one limb (see fig. 4.7). The knack is making sure that the "swing" is controlled enough and does not become a sashay.

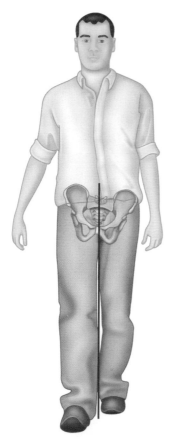

Center of gravity

Figure 4.7. *One of the main strategies the body uses to minimize the effort of bipedal gait is a side swing toward the weight-bearing foot. The combination of this movement and the acceptance of the body weight onto the foot causes the pelvis to drop slightly on the non-weight-bearing side. This passively adducts the hip joint on the weight-bearing side, loading the abductor tissues.*

Following heel strike the greater trochanter shifts laterally into the abductor tissue to stretch the iliotibial band (ITB) from the inside (see fig. 4.7). This tautening of the supportive band of fascia, controlled by the gluteus maximus and gluteus medius (both of which are tensioned to decelerate the flexion and adduction of the hip) and the tensor fasciae latae (tensioned to control adduction) increases the tissue stiffness. Each event assists the other: the contraction of the muscles tightens the fascia, and the tightening of the fascia created by the lateral sway assists the integrity of the muscular contraction.

This combined strategy of shifting the weight to the stance side and allowing the hip joint to adduct reduces the forces that have to be carried by the abductors. This section of tissue works as a "hydraulic amplifier": the fascia lata, stretched tight over the muscles—like shrink wrapping—helps to disperse the force through a greater proportion of tissue (for more, see "Deltoid of the Hip and Hydraulic Amplification" in chapter 5). The sway to the side will push the thigh and pelvis out against the tissue of the abductors, passively increasing the fascial tension throughout the more superficial fascial layers of the thigh and pelvic area on the weight-bearing side. The deeper tissues of the quadriceps and hamstrings expand outward, pressing on the "shrink wrapping" of the fascia lata, and so the area works together, as a system, rather than as individual parts.

The ability to use the ITB in this way develops with age. There is little evidence of an ITB during the time from birth to the early stages of learning to walk. Toddlers tend to walk with a wider stance, flexed hips and knees, and take short steps. Gradually, with increased gait proficiency and practice, the knees move medially to create a valgus angle and bring the feet closer to the midline. These changes are accomplished by an increase in the bicondylar angle (the angle measured between the femoral shaft and the resting plane of its condyles; see fig. 4.8) and through the development of the ITB to provide lateral stability and reinforcement (Cowgill et al. 2010). The increased density of the iliotibial fibers during the toddling phase helps support the underlying femur, which then alters its morphology as the child learns to walk. The femur is thicker medio-laterally in the early years of life up to the early walking phase. As gait matures, the femur thickens in its anterior-posterior axis, with a greater ability to reinforce against sagittal plane forces, while the thicker ITB and stronger abductors now cooperate against medio-lateral forces.

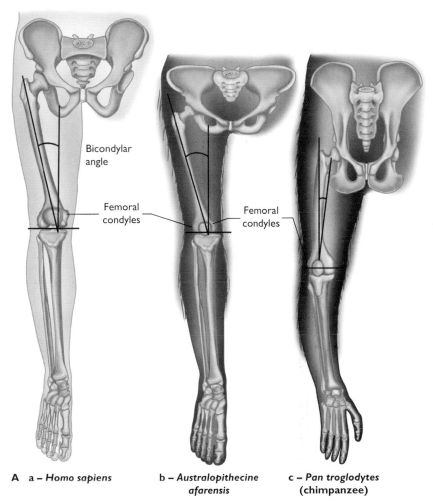

Bicondylar angle

Femoral condyles

Femoral condyles

A   a – Homo sapiens   b – Australopithecine afarensis   c – Pan troglodytes (chimpanzee)

Figure 4.8A. The bicondylar angle of; (a) Homo sapiens, (b) Australopithecine afarensis, (c) chimpanzee. Human legs are less vertically oriented below the hip joint than those of other primates. The increased angle brings our feet closer below our center of gravity and increases the size of the medial condyle – a feature that is developed by walking. (Adapted from Aeillo and Dean 2002.)

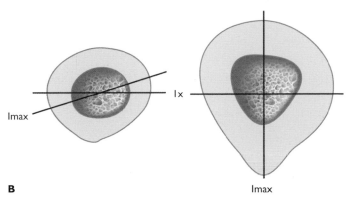

Imax

Ix

B

Imax

Figure 4.8B. Diagram of the mid-shaft femoral cross section of a 2-year-old and a 16-year-old. (From Cowgill et al. 2010.)

Frontal-plane stability is facilitated by the increased bicondylar angle, the anterior-posterior thickening of the femoral mid-shaft, and the development of the ITB. Each of these factors is an indicator of efficient upright gait and can be contrasted with other species (fig. 4.8A; Cowgill et al. 2010, Baker et al. 2011, Eng et al. 2015). The bicondylar angle allows the feet to be positioned more closely below the body's center of mass, but the angle between the hip and the knee requires extra reinforcement from the very strong and elastic ITB, which is much less developed in other species, despite the presence of the attaching muscles (Baker et al. 2011). The human ITB has a variety of muscle attachments to adjust its stiffness, and is generally considered to be continuous with all of the fibers of the tensor fasciae latae, 40–70% of the gluteus maximus (by volume; Eng et al. 2015), and some of the gluteus medius (Baker et al. 2011). The deltoid arrangement of these muscles places them not only as hip abductors but also as flexors and extensors and medial and lateral rotators of the hip. Below, we will explore each aspect of the deltoid in the three planes of movement to fully appreciate their roles in support and movement efficiency.

During the weight acceptance phase, the abdominals provide extra support for the pelvis from above as it tilts down away from the ribs. A contralateral relationship occurs between the lateral abdominals and the opposite hip adductors following heel strike. In fig. 4.7, the iliac crest is moving away from the femur on the right (the heel-strike side), while the ilium and the rib cage are moving away from each other on the left. From a functional point of view, this explains why no evidence of any substantial connection between the gluteus maximus and the same-side abdominals was found by Wilke et al. (2016). The pelvis requires stability from below on the heel-strike side to control hip adduction, and from above on the opposite side to prevent the pelvis dropping too far away from the rib cage during weight transfer. A fascial continuity

between the gluteus maximus and the abdominals might be inefficient in this phase of gait, as it would allow force from one muscle to transfer across the iliac crest on the same side. The pelvis appears to benefit from having contractile forces anchored on either side of the iliac crest to create stability.

This book analyzes each plane of movement in turn, but it is crucial to keep in mind that events coincide in all three planes. For example, the left ilium is supported in all three planes of motion by a variety of tissues (see fig. 4.9). The natural movement of the pelvis, brought about by the action of the lower limbs, creates these lines of tension which are controlled by myofascial tissues. Hopefully, as we add the other lines to the picture, a fully three-dimensional image will come into focus.

■ EFFICIENCY AND THE FEMALE PELVIS

Women have routinely been punished and intimidated for attempting that most simple of freedoms, taking a walk, because their walking and indeed their very beings have been construed as inevitably, continually sexual in those societies concerned with controlling women's sexuality.

—Rebecca Solnit, *Wanderlust: A History of Walking*

There are many restrictive and prejudiced attitudes toward the female pelvis, driven by cultural and religious ideals worldwide, and, sadly, "science" has also jumped on the bandwagon. Since Sherwood Lerned Washburn's usage of the term *obstetric dilemma* (OD) in 1960, there has been a bias toward considering the female pelvis as suffering between two conflicting demands—those of childbirth and those of locomotor efficiency during upright gait. The obstetric dilemma

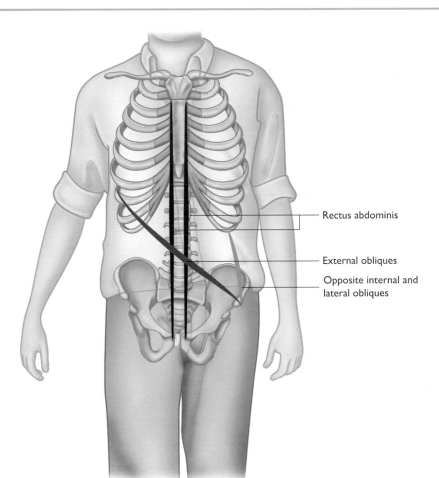

Rectus abdominis

External obliques

Opposite internal and
lateral obliques

Figure 4.9. Following heel strike, the ilium of the opposite limb (shown here as the figure's left side) will be anteriorly and inferiorly tilted and rotated. These movements are controlled/decelerated by the rectus femoris, lateral obliques, and contralateral obliques (external to the opposite internal oblique line shown in red), respectively.

views female pelvic width in a context of directly competing functional requirements: a birth canal wide enough to accommodate the head and body passing through it, and a pelvis narrow enough for locomotor efficiency. A wider canal would require a wider pelvis, and it has been a commonly held belief that a broad pelvis would be biomechanically expensive. Thankfully, recent work has been done to challenge this limited and prejudiced view, which can be questioned on numerous vital assumptions.

Firstly, *Homo sapiens* is not the only species to experience difficult and sometimes dangerous childbirth, so it is not something we have somehow conceded in payment for our upright gait. In a detailed critique of the OD, Helen Dunsworth (2016) points out that spotted hyenas give birth through their clitoris and have an infant mortality rate of 60 percent for first-time mothers. So, as hard as it might be for *Homo sapiens*, it could be worse. Much worse.

Painful, difficult childbirth is not necessarily something that developed as we changed the pelvis for bipedalism. The OD presumes pelvic morphology to have been a compromise between the two demands, as the female pelvis is generally wider than that of the male (fig. 4.10). It is generally true that the medio-lateral measurements between the ischial spines, between the acetabula, and across the pelvic outlet are greater in females than in males, and that this results in a greater valgus angle between the hips and the knees. The wider pelvis has been assumed to be more costly to stabilize, and the increased valgus angle is considered an injury risk. However, counter to common perception, neither pelvic width nor valgus angle negatively affects locomotor efficiency or injury rates.

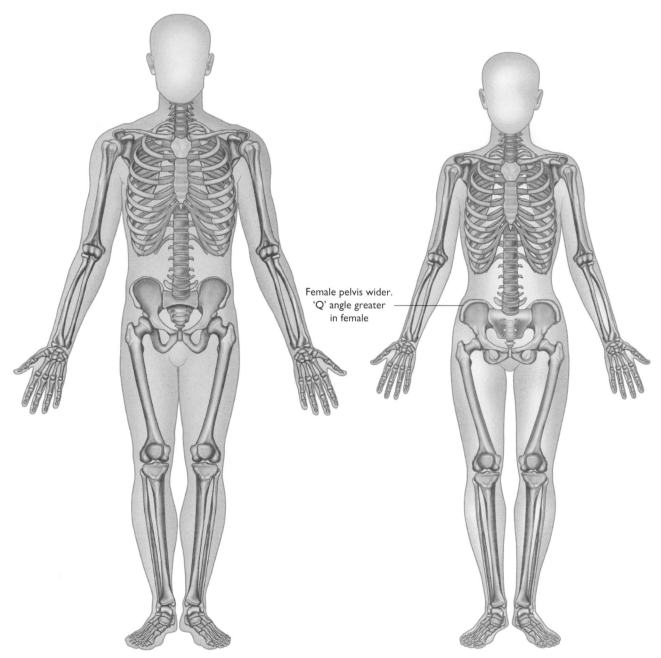

Female pelvis wider. 'Q' angle greater in female

Figure 4.10. Size and shape comparisons of the pelvis between males and females show an overlap, but with a tendency for the female pelvis to be wider and the resultant valgus angle (from hip to knee) to be greater.

Much of the thinking and biomechanical analysis around the OD has been based on static calculations (fig. 4.11A). A study by Warrener et al. (2015) found that when calculations for ground reaction forces and biacetabular width[1] were corrected according to the gait pattern (fig. 4.11B), the results showed parity between male and female subjects and matched their metabolic data measured during walking and running. The results of the study showed "no significant difference in locomotor efficiency between men and women" (Warrener et al. 2015, page 8).

In a further challenge to orthodox thinking, although female athletes are more susceptible

[1]The study showed that a mechanical measurement using the center of the femoral head, rather than the outer surface of the femur (note the differences in placement between fig. 4.10A and B), led to no difference in biacetabular width between male bond female subjects.

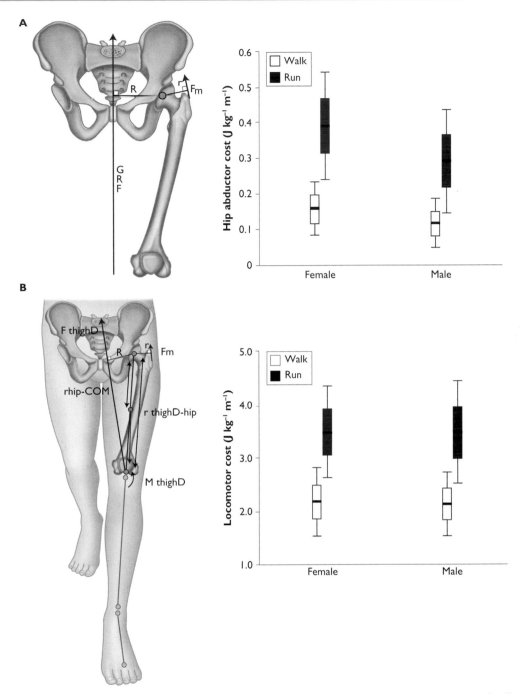

Figure 4.11. *A, Hip abductor costs during locomotion calculated from biomechanical neutral show an increased cost of walking and running for a wider pelvis. B, When calculations are adjusted to replicate the functional positions of the pelvis and femur, there is no significant difference between wide and narrow pelvises for either walking or running. (Adapted from Warrener et al. 2015.)*

to knee injuries (Rozzi et al. 1999) the causes are not solely related to skeletal alignment and valgus angle. Other influencing factors are hormonal differences, higher degrees of joint laxity, and neuromuscular (particularly extensor weakness) differences (Rozzi et al. 1999; Hewett 2006; Powers 2010). Any deficit in these more physiological factors undermines

the stability available for the valgus angle, which is then challenged by the forces involved during movement.

The ITB supports the knee by attaching to Gerdy's tubercle and the tibial tuberosity, especially when the hip adducts and pulls the ITB superiorly and laterally, countering the valgus angle (see fig. 4.11B). As locomotor proficiency develops, it makes sense that the tissue arrangements between soft and skeletal tissues are kept in balance with one another as they respond to biomechanical forces acting through them. Changes in force vectors due to bone growth are optimized by the tissue cells according to Davis' and Wolff's laws (soft tissue and skeletal tissue adapts to mechanical force, respectively). However, these biomechanical laws only apply when all other dynamics for tissue health are functioning; therefore, if there is a weakness in another system, the higher valgus angle for females *does* present an increased potential threat to functional integrity and efficiency.

As we build a better understanding of locomotor mechanics, we may challenge many preconceptions about movement and tissue function. Although research in fascia and elastic dynamics in general has been well established in animal movement, it has been slower to develop in human locomotion. Thankfully, there have been developments in recent years that bode well for future understanding. It just might take a while for the establishment to let go of the obstetric dilemma prejudice.

■ FRONTAL PLANE ADJUSTMENT

Interpreting the EMG readings for the frontal plane muscles is more difficult than for sagittal plane muscles, as each muscle has actions across other the planes. Therefore, we have to analyze their adduction/abduction abilities along with their sagittal and transverse plane actions. A starting point is that the abductors (gluteus maximus upper and lower, TFL, gluteus medius) are firing to help prevent adduction through most of the stance phase (0–62%), with a little preparatory contraction leading up to heel strike from around 90 percent. Except for the TFL, the hip abductors seem to switch off after mid-stance,

when the hip is in sagittal plane neutral, and then remain quiet as the hip passes into extension from 31 percent to 62 percent. We can make sense of this apparent contradiction (the "extensors" are quiet as the hip goes into extension) by remembering the paradox between action and function.

The deltoid arrangement of the hip musculature means that all the abductors and adductors also have flexion and extension abilities. All the muscles behind the frontal plane midline are extensors (such as the gluteus maximus) and those in front are flexors (such as the TFL). From heel strike, the flexed hip must be supported against further flexion, a job that requires the extensors to bring the hip from that position to neutral—the hip is *extending* from the flexed position even if it is not *extended*—and once the hip reaches neutral at mid-stance, the work of the extensors is mostly done. We saw the same thing happen with the hamstrings in the previous chapter (fig. 3.4). Once the hip reaches neutral, momentum should continue to carry the pelvis forward, and the responsibility for control of hip movement passes to the hip flexors—in this case, we see the TFL still working through to 45 percent.

The TFL is active from prior to heel strike as it controls the foot's descent to heel strike, through to early hip extension as the body passes through mid-stance. The TFL therefore appears to control hip extension for a soft heel strike, hip adduction from heel strike to mid-stance, and hip extension from mid-stance to 45 percent. As we saw earlier, it is an important muscle for the control of lower limb stiffness, as it is embedded within the fascia lata of the thigh, along with the superior portion of gluteus maximus. In fact, as we will see later, these two muscles may be better viewed as anterior and posterior portions of the same muscle—the deltoid of Farabeuf (see "Deltoid of the Hip and Hydraulic Amplification" in chapter 5; fig. 5.8).

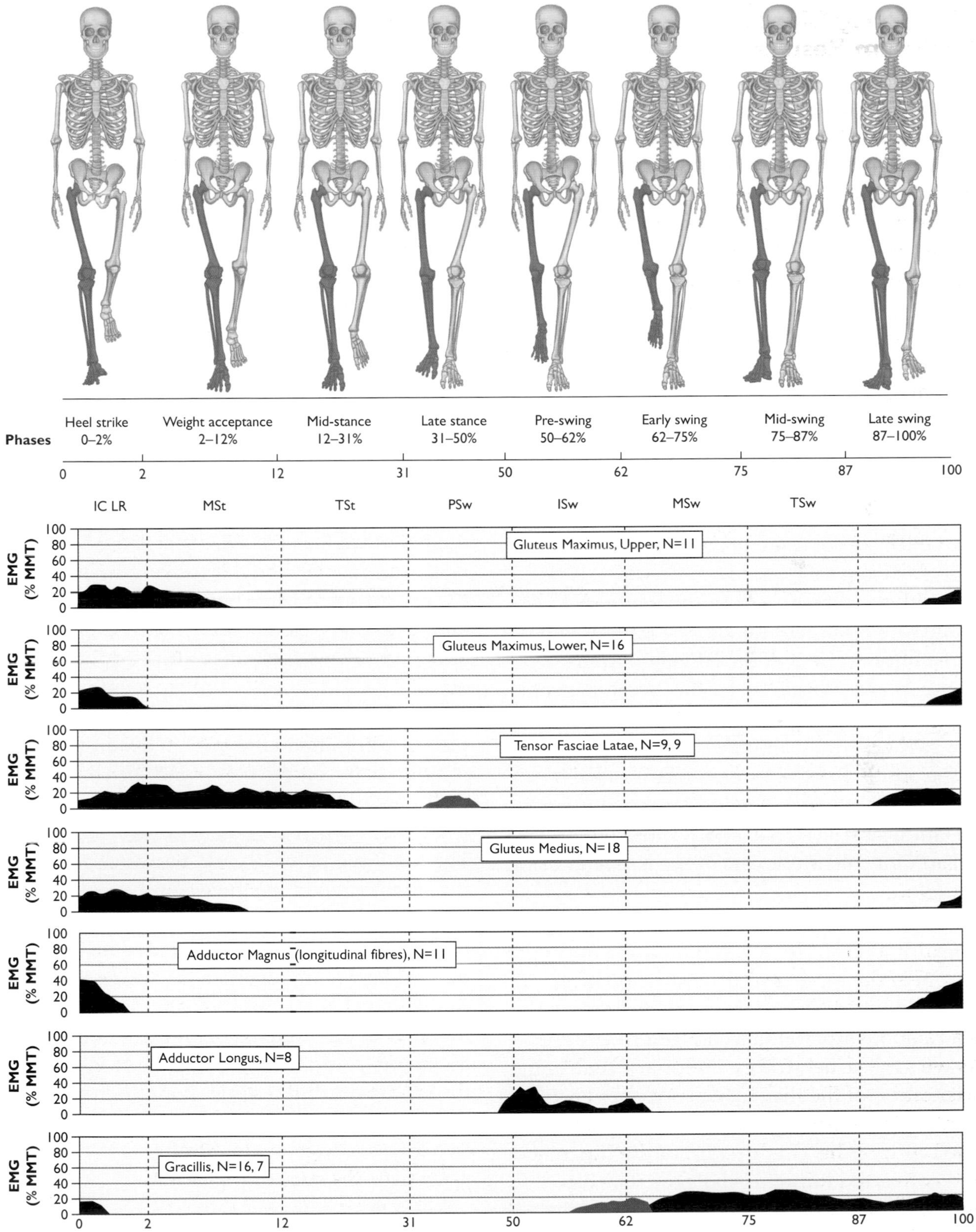

Figure 4.12. *The frontal plane gait cycle. (Adapted from Perry and Burnfield 2010.)*

Minimizing Effort for Maximum Results

When we look at the EMG readings for the gluteus maximus, it seems that this muscle makes very little effort in the control of flexion and adduction. There are two aspects to be aware of—firstly, it is a powerful muscle and the figures are a percentage of maximum muscle tension, so a small contraction of a strong muscle can still be quite a lot of force. Secondly, and importantly for this text, we have to ensure that we optimize the pre-tension of the connective tissue around the gluteus maximus by enabling an appropriate range of motion in each plane—i.e., enough hip flexion, hip adduction, and medial rotation—to allow this muscle to be more effective at controlling each of those movements.

The interrelationships between joints and tissues are relatively easy to see in the sagittal plane but require a different vision in the frontal plane. We analyzed the essential events for the sagittal plane in the previous chapter and saw how they all influence the length of the stride. If we shorten the stride, we lose some of the pre-tension for the gluteus maximus at heel strike, and we lose the pre-tension for the hip flexors of the back hip prior to toe-off.

Recruiting the abductors as extensors and flexors of the hip is simply a function of the angles at which the fibers cross the joint and is a relationship that has changed over time. As we saw earlier, the evolutionary change in orientation of the iliac blades not only enabled frontal plane loading during stance phase but also brought the TFL forward of the hip joint and converted it into a hip flexor. The hip abductor deltoid is now able to support the hip joint in each plane as it progresses through flexion to extension and through lateral to medial rotation during the stance phase.

The stance phase requires the ability to displace the body weight over the supporting foot to realign the center of gravity, and the hip should be able to adduct by approximately 4 degrees. The ability to achieve a 4-degree tilt will pre-tension the gluteus maximus (and the other abductors) in the frontal plane; the opposite adductors and lateral abdominals will also have to lengthen for the tilt to occur. The tilt of the pelvis can therefore be hindered by many other factors, each of which could functionally "weaken" the gluteus maximus by reducing the amount of pre-tension.

The pelvic tilt also helps align the center of gravity over the feet, which is also facilitated by the bicondylar angle discussed earlier. The bicondylar angle requires a medial femoral condyle that is larger than the lateral one, and this allows them both to rest securely on the tibial plateau (see fig. 4.8A; see also fig. 1.8A). Because of the bicondylar (or valgus) angle, the abductors must be both strong enough to deal with body weight and able to lengthen enough to allow the transfer and adduction to occur. The adduction of the hip lengthens the abdominals on the opposite side in the frontal plane, aiding their efficiency in dealing with the rotation between the pelvis and the rib cage, as well as with the drop of the pelvis.

The tilt of the pelvis should be absorbed by the side flexion of the lower lumbar spine (S1–L3), otherwise the lateral deviation will be sent to the thoracolumbar junction, causing overextension and overuse (as addressed in the "Clinical Note" below). Any decreased mobility in the lumbars or stiffness in the hip abductors could lead to upper body sway, as the client will find it difficult to differentiate between the pelvis and the rib cage, causing the two to move together and bringing the whole body over the supporting foot.

Earlier we explored the role of the ITB as a stabilizer of knee valgus because of the bicondylar angle, but we also need to view it as the extended tendon of the gluteus maximus (a hip extensor), and the TFL (a hip flexor)—collectively, the deltoid of the hip abductors.

The posterior and anterior portions of the ITB will therefore be tensioned by hip position and the resultant contraction of these muscles at either end of their range, which happens at heel strike and toe-off. Ground reaction force is at its peak through heel strike and early weight acceptance (see fig. 2.13), and a long moment arm[2] exists between the body's center of mass and the foot's point of contact with the ground. The position of heel strike creates a number of offset forces in the sagittal and frontal planes, each of which must be controlled or the body will otherwise collapse to some degree. The gluteus maximus (along with the other hip extensors) will have to contract to control further flexion of the hip because of the offset between the body's mass and the support coming up from the ground. It makes sense that the forward swing of the leg pre-tensions the extensors (better thought of in this case as the decelerators of flexion!) in preparation for the load they are about to receive at heel strike.

Frontal Plane Meets Sagittal Plane

Only the upper fibers of the gluteus maximus are continuous with the posterior ITB, and we see them contracting through the mid-stance phase. The gluteus maximus is therefore active from the moment the hip is flexed prior to heel strike until it passes neutral and goes into extension. The gluteus maximus is then quiescent during late stance and toe-off, which is when the TFL and other hip flexors are more important for deceleration as the forward momentum of the pelvis begins to tension and load the anterior tissues.

A study by Eng and colleagues (2015) explored this deltoid arrangement between the TFL and the gluteus maximus around the hip during

running. They were able to demonstrate that the gluteus maximus–ITB pair is maximally tensioned at late swing, when the hip is flexed, and that the TFL ITB pair is maximally tensioned during early swing because of the hip extension during running. The study found significant energy is transmitted along the ITB during running, and though the forces would be smaller, it is still likely that the ITB will be involved in energy transmission in the sagittal plane as well as the frontal plane during normal walking.

Eng's research shows similar findings to our exploration of the flexors and extensors in the previous chapter: there needs to be a long enough stride for the ITB to achieve some degree of force transmission. Furthermore, for frontal plane stability, the hip also needs to adduct to add pre-tension to the lateral hip tissues. Fig. 4.12 shows another hip abductor, the gluteus medius, helping control the adduction moment in the frontal plane as we progress through stance. As the forward hip adducts during the early stance period the pelvis begins to tilt, which requires a reciprocal abduction of the opposite hip. An interdependent and contralateral relationship therefore exists between the hip abductors on one side and the adductors on the opposite side, as both groups have to lengthen to optimize tissue tensioning in the frontal plane and to facilitate weight transfer to the forward limb during the weight acceptance phase.

It is possible that the interdependency between the hip abductors and the opposite hip adductors can be a cause of dysfunction. Commonly, the gluteus maximus is blamed for the lack of control of the lower limb following heel strike, but it may not be the gluteal tissue that is at fault. Many tissues have to cooperate to allow the pelvis to tilt and the gluteus maximus to pre-tension, such as when there is an inability to open the anterior adductors of the opposite hip. To fully explore dynamic hip ability, the clinician should consider checking

[2]A moment arm is used here to signify the distance between the two forces (ground reaction force at the point of heel strike and momentum within the body's center of mass), which create a simple lever mechanic. I have used *moment* here to avoid giving the impression of levers in our anatomy.

at least three areas—the hip abductors, the hip adductors, and the lower lumbar spine (see fig. 4.13).

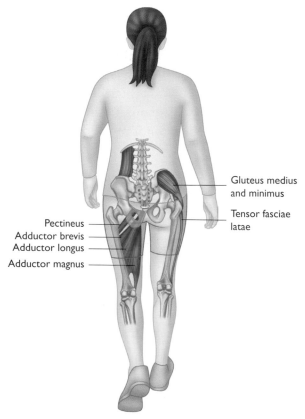

Figure 4.13. *The side sway and hip adduction following heel strike requires at least three areas of adaptation. The hip abductors on the forward limb must lengthen to allow the pelvis to drop, an action also facilitated by the hip adductors on the other leg. If the pelvis tilts, the lower lumbars should be able to absorb some of that movement in its lower section to remove some stress from the thoracolumbar junction. The lumbar movement will be controlled by the iliolumbar fibers of the quadratus lumborum, but it could also be influenced by overly taught lateral abdominals. This triad of soft tissue is arranged in a triangular pattern.*

The EMG readings provide us with data from only a few of the adductors, but we see an interesting dynamic between the hip flexor adductor (adductor longus), the midline adductor (gracilis), and the extensor adductor (adductor magnus)—a similar deltoid-like arrangement to the one we saw for the abductors. Fig. 4.12 shows that the adductor longus fires from before toe-off (decelerating the final moments of hip extension) to mid-swing (when the hip is neutral in the sagittal plane), and then switches off as the hip goes into

extension. The gracilis is active from late stance to heel strike, probably because the forward swing causes the pelvis to rotate away from the advancing limb and this must be decelerated from the inside of the hip. Being so close to the frontal plane midline allows the gracilis to assist with the control of both flexion and extension, as well as abduction during the swing phase. The more specialized adductor magnus is only active either side of heel strike. As a strong hip extensor and adductor, the adductor magnus will contract to decelerate and control the flexion and abduction in the latter stages of the swing phase and prepare for the stronger work of controlling those same movements in the moments following heel strike.

■ ESSENTIAL EVENTS

Side Flexion of the Lumbar Spine

The tilt of the pelvis helps to stimulate the abdominals, and it also requires an adaptation in the spine. If we look at the lateral flexion ability of each segment of the spine on the spinal movement chart (fig. 4.14), we see that the lower lumbars have a gradual increase in lateral flexibility up to L3/L4.

The side flexion of the lowest lumbars lets the spine briefly mimic a tree growing on a hillside. The lower part of the trunk will adapt its growth to send the rest of the tree skyward (see fig. 4.15A). The lower lumbar area absorbs the frontal plane movement of the pelvis, with the iliolumbar fibers of the quadratus lumborum correcting the tilt of the pelvis and the iliolumbar ligament preventing further hip adduction (see fig. 4.15B). If this system loses some of its adaptability, the tilt may be forced up to the thoracolumbar junction, which also allows side flexion (see fig. 4.14), before reaching the vertebrae of the less flexible thoracic cage.

The images used here present a simplified model of spinal motion taken from the

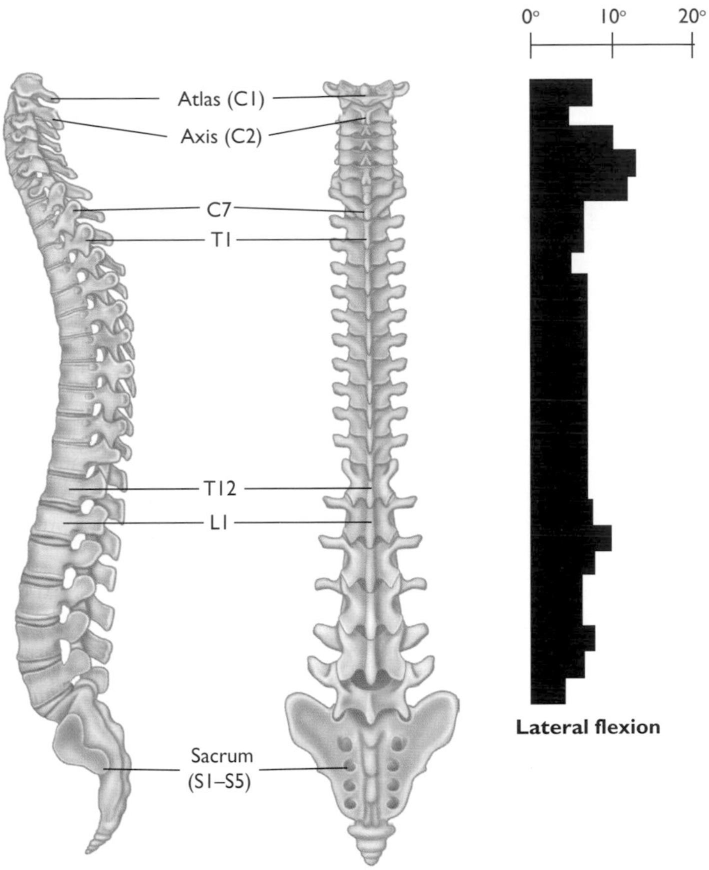

Figure 4.14. *For head stability, the spine must adapt to and diminish movement in the three planes of movement occurring in the pelvis. Much of the lateral tilt (a frontal plane movement) is dealt with by the lower lumbars, L3 and below. The chart shows a gradual increase in side flexion ability from L5/S1 up to L3/L4, a slight decrease in the mid-lumbars, and another increase around the thoracolumbar junction. Side flexion ability stays relatively consistent throughout the thoracics until the cervicothoracic junction. (Adapted from Middleditch and Oliver 2005.)*

anatomical position. Spinal movement during gait is in reality too complex for an exploration in this short text to do it justice. Facet joint alignment through the spine means that certain motions are naturally coupled, and, as such, side flexion of the lumbars will automatically create rotation through them as well. The degrees of movement shown in fig. 4.14 can also increase or decrease depending on the amount of flexion or extension the spine is positioned in. (To gain a more complete picture of spinal movement, the dedicated therapist is recommended to explore this further[3].) It remains true, however, that lumbar side flexion is an essential event, because not only does it allow the abductors and opposite adductors to work appropriately, but it also couples the spine into rotation to assist the spinal muscles, especially the multifidi (Gracovetsky 2008).

Clinical Note

A simple test for the ability of the pelvis to drop away from the lower lumbars rather than the upper ones is to have your client stand in front of you and bend one knee. Ask him or her to keep both feet on the floor, and the foot on the target side will naturally roll forward on the ankle or forefoot rocker (see fig. 4.16A). This will cause the pelvis to drop on one side, and the bend should occur predominantly in the section of the spine below L3 (see fig. 4.16B).

[3]Although it may require some degree of pre-study, Serge Gracovetsky's "Spinal Engine" is a detailed exploration of spinal mechanics during gait. Introductory lectures on his spinal engine model can also be found online.

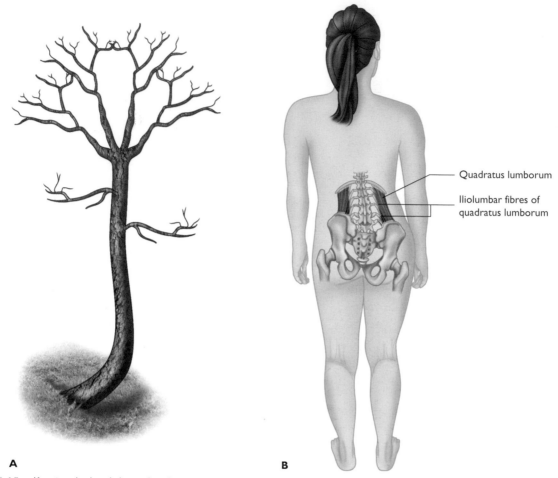

A   **B**

Quadratus lumborum

Iliolumbar fibres of
quadratus lumborum

Figure 4.15. Keeping the head skyward and minimizing its tilt requires a reduction of the adduction that occurs at the hip in natural gait. Like the bend of the tree trunk (A), most of the deviation of the pelvis in frontal plane movement can be absorbed low down in the spine if the movement is allowed by the iliolumbar ligaments and the iliolumbar fibers of the quadratus lumborum (B). If it is not, the side flexion will travel higher (as we saw with the rotation) and can create—or demand—a hypermobility around the thoracolumbar junction.

Hip Adduction and Opposite Hip Abduction for Weight Transfer

Stride length in the sagittal plane naturally leads to a tilt of the pelvis. As the forward leg swings, the pelvis tilts toward the back stance limb. The tilt is dependent on hip adduction on the swing side and abduction on the stance side, and is allowed by side flexion in the lower lumbars. A number of factors can prevent or inhibit the ability to properly adduct the forward limb, and failure to do so may lead to the presentation of a number of clinical issues.

The gluteus maximus is especially involved in the control of knee valgus, a work load that is eased if its tissue is allowed to lengthen before the shock of heel strike. As we saw above, the increased valgus angle common among females is only a problem if other factors are not working correctly. One of those factors is the biomechanical relationships around the pelvis. To fully assist the loading of the gluteus maximus to control the valgus angle, the functional triangle of the abductors, opposite adductors, and lumbar side flexors must behave appropriately, and can be easily tested for both range of motion and strength using some of the suggestions above (fig. 4.16) in association with any good orthopedic assessment guide. A few further suggestions are also outlined for you below.

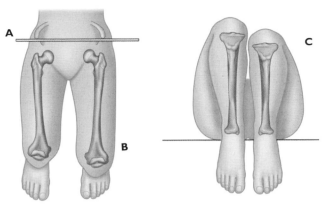

Figure 4.17. *In this standard orthopedic test, ensure that both anterior superior iliac spines (ASIS) are level and place the medial malleoli together to create a neutral position (A). This will allow the therapist to assess the length of the femurs and the heights of the tibia. A longer femur will reveal itself by pushing the knee further from the body (B), and a longer tibia will produce a higher tibial tuberosity or knee-joint line (C). It is important for the feet to be placed parallel to the pelvis and in the midline in order to read the legs in an anatomical neutral.*

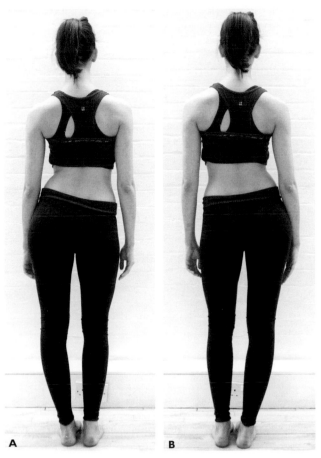

Figure 4.16. *Ask your client to stand with feet hip-width apart and roughly parallel, and then simply bend one knee, keeping the foot on the floor (A). This will cause the pelvis to drop on the side of the bent knee, and the freedom of the lumbars on the opposite side can be assessed. A responsive spine will show a clear lateral bend before L3 (B); a spine that is unable to absorb the movement in the lower lumbars will force the bend to occur higher in the spine.*

Leg-Length Differences

Leg-length differences can affect the movements of the pelvis. The client can be assessed by placing the medial malleoli together and having his or her knees bent. In this position, any structural length differences in the tibia or femur will be apparent (see fig. 4.17).

Any discrepancy in leg length may be compensated for by changes in the arches—the long leg may pronate or the shorter one supinate, or sometimes there may be a combination of the two—and these alterations can effectively balance the limbs. This can

have implications for therapeutic input, as the compensations may be beneficial for the client. Thus, any work with the feet should also address the rest of the system to ensure that it is able to cope with the new positions.

Foot Balance

Changes in the feet can also lead to "apparent" differences in leg length. The lower limb may appear longer if the foot is more supinated, or it can appear shorter if the foot is pronated. These cases of functional leg-length difference may be easier to correct than dealing with real length differences, which will require a more detailed understanding of the many compensations that may have occurred in the client's body. Each case will require individual recommendations, but we will explore some options in the next couple of chapters.

Structural Shifts

A longer leg can create an angled sacral base, which the spine must adapt to by bending to one side. If the body is held long enough in a shifted position, it may adapt to that pattern by creating restricted or adhered tissue (fig. 4.18). A slight deviation in the lower spine can develop when a parent frequently carries his or her child on a raised hip, or if a person who drives for long periods sits with one hip raised on an angled car seat or with a wallet in the back pocket. This displacing of the body weight to one side may lead to further frontal plane discrepancies in movement, and/or create limitations in gait because of restricted tissue.

Bends in the spine may also lead to restricted movement in the spinal facets, especially in the transverse plane. The closing of the articulations on one side of the vertebral column in the frontal plane will affect the

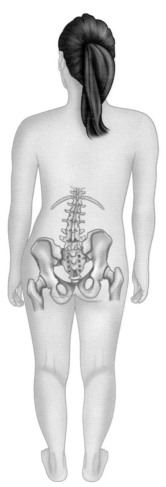

Figure 4.18. *Having the sacral base angled to one side will create lateral bends in the spine. These can lead to tissue restrictions, especially around the iliolumbar ligament and the lower fibers of the quadratus lumborum, and it may restrict the facet joint movement in the other planes.*

spine's ability to rotate, which can lead to many potential compensations—shorter strides, overextension in other spinal segments, or a lumbering side-to-side gait, as described above. Dealing with the structural issues first by easing the side bends before dealing with the functional issues can therefore be an appropriate strategy.[4]

■ SUMMARY

1. The laterally facing ilia and the valgus and bicondylar angles all allow foot placement closer to the midline during stance phase.
2. Laterally facing ilia provide attachment for an abductor deltoid that controls adduction as well as sagittal and transverse plane movements.
3. We naturally swing our pelvis to the side of the stance leg, bringing our center of gravity over the base of support—the stance foot—and minimizing the work of maintaining balance.
4. The movement of the pelvis and resultant adduction of the hip help to load the myofascial tissue of the abductors on the stance leg, as well as the opposite-side adductors, quadratus lumborum, and abdominals, thereby increasing efficiency and assisting with the recoil back to neutral.
5. Pelvic tilt can be inhibited by many factors (including cultural and emotional), and time should be spent testing each of the essential events—same-side hip abductors, opposite-side hip adductors, and lower lumbar side flexors.
6. The essential events that allow us to take advantage of frontal plane efficiency mechanisms are: lumbar side flexion, hip adduction of the stance limb, and hip abduction of the opposite limb.

This chapter has shown the benefits and the potential restrictors of side-to-side pelvic tilt.

---

[4]For full descriptions on how to do this, see Earls and Myers, *Fascial Release for Structural Balance* (2017).

There is a complex interplay between the abductors and opposite adductors of the hip, which should coincide with lower lumbar side flexion. If each of these areas is strong enough to control and absorb the 4-degree tilt of the pelvis, then the load of the lateral tissues helps to regulate the pronation cascade following heel strike. It is a complex and multi-dimensional action which should not really be divided up into separate units—the pelvis tilts and the hip tissues (left and right), abdominals, and lower back muscles all cooperate simultaneously. The sequence is only broken down here because language forces us to do so.

The importance of pelvic tilt was highlighted by the recent research of Warrener et al. (2015), which showed that tilting balanced out any potential biomechanical issues caused by a wider pelvis—driving another nail into the coffin of the sexist ideas around the obstetric dilemma. Their results also highlighted the benefits of letting movement happen and not maintaining "pelvic stability"—allowing the pelvis to swing enough and not too much gives many efficiency benefits.

5

TRANSVERSE PLANE

Do not all charms fly
At the mere touch of cold philosophy?
There was an awful rainbow
once in heaven:
We know her woof, her texture;
she is given
In the dull catalogue of common things.
Philosophy will clip an Angel's wings,
Conquer all mysteries by rule and line,
Empty the haunted air, and
gnomèd mine—
Unweave a rainbow, as it erewhile made
The tender-person'd Lamia melt
into a shade.

—John Keats, "To Science."

■ INTRODUCTION

Keats' poem alerts us to the threat of losing the beauty of the natural world by explaining it with science. Like many other responses since then, I hope to show that understanding the reality is even more wondrous than the myths of movement that are sometimes held.

The transverse plane is key to understanding gait. Rotational forces are omnipresent during walking, as they are caused by offset bones and offset forces. As we saw with the abductors in the frontal plane, all muscles have the potential for movement control in each plane, and we will explore areas where the muscles appear to cooperate along tensional lines.

In the first edition of this book, I used Myers' Spiral Line as the model to describe movement regulation in the transverse plane, but I have moved away from this, as the Spiral Line is rarely tensioned along its full length. However, despite its myofascial continuity being challenged (Wilke et al. 2016), we will see that the fascicular direction of the Spiral Line tissue does match a line of strain created at toe-off.

The transverse plane returns us to the foot and its capacity to pronate and supinate. From heel strike to mid-stance we have to control the pronation cascade and then supinate the foot again between mid-stance and toe-off. Pronation sends a rotation response up the lower limb, and a counterrotation after mid-stance then helps it supinate and stabilize before toe-off. The counterrotation comes down the limb to the foot because of the turning of the pelvis as its responds to the forward swing of the other leg.

In chapter 3 we saw that pelvic rotation contributed to stride length and was created by the offset between the tensioning hip flexors on one side and the extensors on the other as one leg swings forward. Pelvic rotation also causes oblique tension through the trunk and into the shoulder girdle to create a watch spring–like mechanism. The watch spring contributes a transverse plane catapult when the system is appropriately wound up.

The essential events for the transverse plane are pronation and supination of the foot, mobility of the sacroiliac joints, thoracic rotation, and contralateral arm swing.

Econcentricity
(with thanks and credit to the Gray Institute)

First, we have to clarify the different types of tensioning that can occur at various phases. Muscles can contract concentrically and eccentrically, but—somewhat confusingly— they can also apparently lengthen at one end or in one plane and shorten at the other (Gray and Tiberio refer to this as *econcentric*). In this "econcentric" contraction, the muscle fiber is often acting predominantly isometrically, and the movement of one bone (i.e., at one end of the muscle) is drawing the end of the muscle along with it. We see this in the tensor fasciae latae, which will "lengthen" with hip extension but simultaneously "shorten" as a result of the internal rotation of the hip as we progress toward the toe-off position. Breaking away from the eccentric/concentric model in this way allows us to see tissue interaction more clearly and not just in a binary—lengthening or shortening—vocabulary.

Looking at the muscles in this way, we can see that they are not only actively working (i.e., contracting), but also adjusting the stiffness held within the system. Through experience, our bodies learn to sense the ideal level of tension that facilitates the correct movement sequence and utilize momentum from distant body parts to assist energy efficiency. The muscles are therefore tensioners within a "stiffness-adjusting system," fine-tuning the correct amount of tension by either "gathering in" (concentric contraction) or "letting out" (eccentric contraction) in relation to the events all around and allowing as much loading into the elastic fascial tissue as possible.

In chapter 3 we saw how the work of Sawicki and others points toward the muscles' ability to constantly attune to the various forces surrounding them. Gravity, ground reaction force, and momentum all have to be contextualized within the natural stiffness of the tissues involved in the movement. For example, in a situation of high momentum, a long slender tendon with less stiffness may need to be "drawn" in by a concentric contraction to help stabilize the movement. Conversely, a muscle with short tendons under low stress may need to be "let out" to allow movement to happen. The ideal is where there is an optimal balance between the repeated forces normally experienced by the tissues and the length and elasticity of the tendons. This allows the associated muscle to remain closer to an isometric contraction. We saw the expression of this dynamic in chapter 1 when looking at the different myofascial unit architectures of the sartorius, gastrocnemius, and semimembranosus.

In this chapter, we again see the important contribution of the mechanoreceptors embedded within the soft tissue: how they sense tension, movement, and shearing and relay this information to the surrounding tissue, striving for optimal efficiency.

Chapter 2 outlined the sequence of events following heel strike—a complex cascade of events taking place in all three planes of motion. So far, we have dealt with the sagittal and frontal planes, and now it is the turn (if you will excuse the pun) of the transverse plane. The rotation will switch on the body's obliquely oriented fibers, many of which we have already explored. The transverse plane

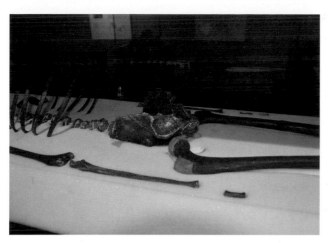

Figure 5.1. *The long waist—seen here in the remains of "Turkana Boy," found in Kenya and dated to 1.5 MYA—shows the potential for counterrotation between the pelvis and the rib cage. Counterrotation is rarely seen in nonhuman primates, because of the shorter distance between these two body segments.*

overlap with other tissues should not surprise us: our increased use of transverse plane movement is a relatively new adaptation, one enhanced in our primate heritage by the development of a long waist approximately 1.5 million years ago, first seen in fossils of *Homo ergaster* (fig. 5.1).

The many evolutionary changes in our skeletal structure were concomitant with changes in the alignment of our musculature. The actual muscles themselves did not change—it was simply their actions and functions that changed as they adapted to the new pathways forged within whichever skeletal "river beds" they ran through. Therefore, the development of the arch of the foot, the closer alignment of the big toe, the angulation of the femurs, and the relative independence between the thoracic cage and the pelvis introduced more rotation and allowed the musculature to act in all three planes.

■ A REMINDER ON REAL AND RELATIVE MOTION

Transverse plane mechanics can be confusing until one is familiar with real and relative motion, or osteokinematics and

arthrokinematics (introduced in chapter 2). When looking at fig. 5.2, we see the series of medial rotations of the tibia and femur following heel strike, and it makes sense to us that the "knee" is also medially rotating. The knee is considered to be medially rotated because the distal bone (the tibia) is moving further than the proximal bone (the femur), and a similar event is happening at the hip joint. Although the hip is laterally rotated at heel strike, the femur medially rotates below it (0–2% of the gait cycle), and so the joint will be medially rotating.

Following toe-off of the opposite limb, the swing leg progresses in front of the body and pulls the pelvis toward the stance foot (31–62%). Therefore, from mid-stance to toe-off, the reaction through the stance limb is driven from the pelvis downward, whereas following heel strike, the reaction travels up from the calcaneus and talus. The change in direction is critical in understanding what is happening across the joints.

Between mid-stance and toe-off, the bones of the stance limb will laterally rotate, but we see the pelvis turn more than the femur, creating medial rotation at the hip. The turning of the pelvis encourages the femur to rotate laterally more than the tibia, which also creates medial rotation at the knee. Therefore, medial rotation of the knee occurs at either end of the stance period—following heel strike and in preparation for toe-off. The alignment of the cruciate ligaments at the knee, as seen in fig. 2.30, allows the coupling at the knee joint to accommodate either a bottom-up or a top-down driven movement of the bones.

The coupling dynamic facilitated by the cruciate ligaments across the knee joint allows the turning of the pelvis toward the stance leg to laterally rotate the tibial and fibular malleoli to assist the form closure of the foot in preparation for toe-off. The turning of the pelvis is driven by the leg swing, which is tied to the

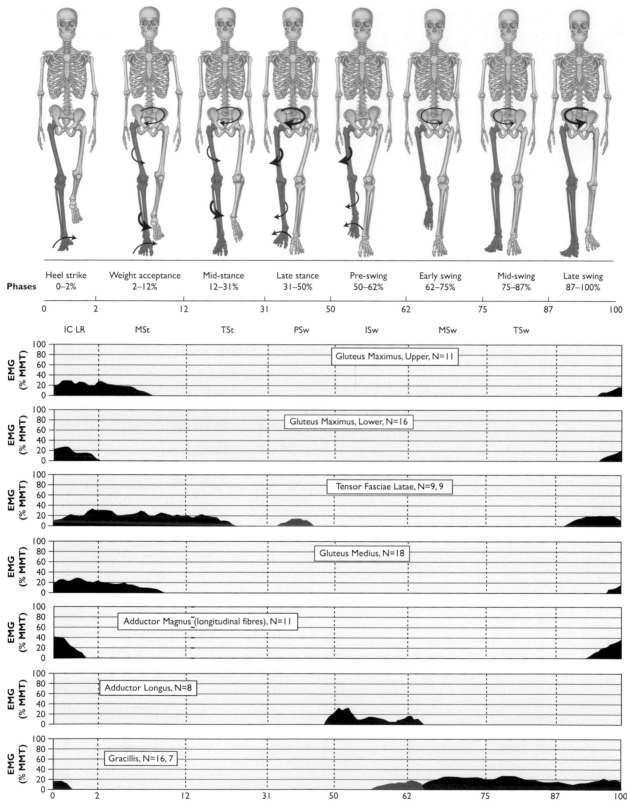

Figure 5.2. *Many changes occur throughout the gait cycle in the transverse plane. The offset of the calcaneus and the talus initiates the unlocking of the tarsal bones and drives rotation up the associated limb following heel strike (0–31%), and the forward swing of the opposite limb drives an opposite rotation down the stance leg to re-supinate the foot in preparation for toe-off (31–62%). After toe-off, the swing of the leg creates a rotation away from the forward limb to assist the supination of the other foot (62–100%). The rotation of the pelvis, driven by the lower limbs, creates a relative rotation between it and the rib cage to lengthen the abdominals and intercostals as the arms serve to counterbalance the rotational force from above. (Adapted from Perry and Burnfield 2010.)*

length of the stride and is therefore influenced by all of the essential events explored in chapter 3. However, the loss of any sagittal plane essential event can lead to increased rotation of the pelvis as a compensation for loss of stride length, but it will be driven by the torso rather than the leg swing and will have a noticeably more effortful character.

To grasp the idea of real and relative motion, it is important to be rigorous with the naming of the bones and joints. Much confusion is caused by loose terminology and by only looking at one aspect—the bone or the joint—during movement. Being able to visualize both types of movement—real and relative—assists one's mental picture of force transfer and coupling through the system.

■ LOWER LIMB MECHANICS

Calcaneal Eversion/Inversion and the Ankle Rocker

The best place to start our exploration of transverse plane movement during gait is from the moment of heel strike. We looked at the evolution and functional ability of the foot's half-dome in chapter 2 and saw how the offset between the calcaneus and the talus (and therefore the offset between ground reaction forces and the body's momentum) creates calcaneal eversion. Eversion of the heel bone sets up a sequence of rotations that unlocks the midtarsal bones distally and sends a medial rotation of the tibia, fibula, and femur up the lower limb.

Unlocking the mid-foot opens the joints and allows the plantar tissues to absorb the shock. The freedom of the joints allows the foot to mold to the surface during the early to mid-stance phases, after which it must come back to a close-packed position to form a rigid lever. The stability of the rigid lever is necessary in order to create a stable platform for energy

release at toe-off. This unlocking and locking dynamic is primarily managed through the bones using transverse plane coupling for "form opening and closing," but will also involve a significant number of soft tissues to assist "force closure" of the foot and ankle complex. As we saw in the sagittal and frontal planes, both of these closure dynamics require appropriate ranges of motion in each associated joint and soft tissue.

The fibulares evert the calcaneus and could be involved in force opening of the foot. Myers (2015) suggests that the ITB is continuous with the fibulares as part of the Lateral Line (see fig. 5.3), and in chapter 4 we saw the deltoid of the hip (and therefore the ITB) tension during weight acceptance. In the EMG readings, we do not see the fibulares responding until after mid-stance, when they must control ankle dorsiflexion and lengthen to allow the foot to correct itself back to supination in preparation for toe-off. As the limb progresses through the ankle and foot rockers (see figs. 5.4 to 5.6), the dorsiflexion and toe extension will require the tissue of both fibularis muscles to be free from tethering (i.e., each must be free to glide through its associated retinaculum), and to be long enough

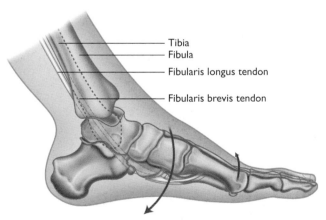

Figure 5.3. *Any force that comes along the fascia of the ITB and into the fascial tissue of the fibularis longus and brevis may help the foot adapt to the ground. The fibularis longus may help the medial tilt of the medial cuneiform and first metatarsal, while the fibularis brevis may encourage the forefoot to laterally rotate, via its insertion into the base of the fifth metatarsal.*

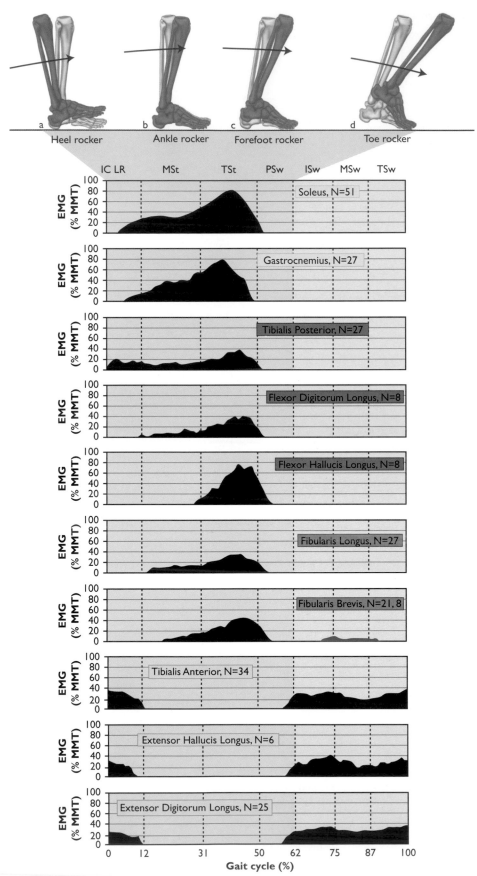

Figure 5.4. *EMG readings for the leg muscles during gait. (Adapted from Perry and Burnfield 2010.)*

for the medial arch to lift again, which will allow the forefoot to come back in line with the calcaneus (see fig. 5.5).

In early mid-stance, the EMG readings show a switch between the anterior compartment (tibialis anterior and long toe extensors), the only dorsiflexors, and the ankle plantar flexor groups (see fig. 5.4). At mid-stance, the ankle moves from being plantar flexed into dorsiflexion, and the plantar flexors are recruited to decelerate the forward momentum. Their tensioning also assists with the foot's force closing to supination. During gait, the plantar flexors predominantly work eccentrically, in contrast to the dorsiflexors of the anterior compartment. The muscles of the anterior compartment contract from pre-swing all the way through to mid-stance to provide foot clearance. Drawing the foot up during the swing phase requires an active concentric contraction of this group until heel strike, when they must eccentrically control plantar flexion following the heel rocker at landing. Without the eccentric control from the tibialis anterior and the long toe extensors, the foot would slap down after heel strike. The same muscles then stay active during weight acceptance to further assist control of pronation. The pronation response is also controlled by the tibialis posterior, which fires immediately on heel strike (fig. 5.4), well before the other plantar flexors.

A restriction of the ankle rocker, whether due to a block of the anterior joint or a constriction of the Achilles tendon or posterior compartments, can lead to an exaggerated gait with the toes pointed out. Differential diagnosis of some form is required to find the culprit; often it is due to the commonly overlooked fibularis compartment. Whether or not the fibularis muscles were the original cause, if the foot is not combining dorsiflexion with inversion, these muscles may not get challenged to their end of range and may develop a functional shortness, thereby becoming part of the problem. Exercises and stretches that combine dorsiflexion with

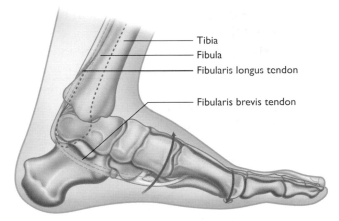

Tibia
Fibula
Fibularis longus tendon
Fibularis brevis tendon

Figure 5.5. Once the ankle comes into dorsiflexion, the foot must be assisted back to its neutral position from its pronated position. This supination of the foot requires lengthening of the fibularis tissue to bring the foot back from the lateral rotation and medial tilt. The fascia of the fibulares is able to relax as the strain transferred down from the hip abductors is gradually unloaded by the body first coming into line above the foot and then heel striking on the opposite side.

inversion should be included in most foot and ankle routines (if safe to do so).

The fibulares are essential for correct functioning of the foot's medial aspect. The fibularis longus is required to draw the first metatarsal into the medial cuneiform, while the fibularis brevis performs a similar role for the fifth metatarsal. If the fibularis brevis is unable to lengthen fully as the ankle dorsiflexes, it will keep the foot in a laterally rotated position, which often prevents the midtarsal joints from reengaging prior to toe-off (see fig. 2.16). We see this in fig. 5.4, where both the invertors (tibialis posterior and flexors hallucis and digitorum longus) and the evertors (fibularis brevis and longus) of the ankle are contracting as the ankle dorsiflexes between mid-stance and toe-off. It is necessary for the two muscle groups to be in balance in order to allow correct alignment and correction of the foot prior to toe-off.

Control of the Pronation Cascade

The sequence of events following the pronation of the foot has to be decelerated and controlled. Once the talus medially rotates and tilts on top of the calcaneus, it will bring the tibia and therefore the femur along with it, creating strong rotational forces at the joints (see chapter 2). If we follow the line of force along the lower limb, we come to the gluteus maximus and the ITB (see fig. 5.6). Myers (2015) suggests the ITB to be part of a continuity from the TFL to the tibialis anterior, but in this phase of gait, it makes more sense to use a continuity from the gluteus maximus to the tibialis anterior via the ITB, as both muscles appear to have a similar firing pattern and fascicular direction to enable control of the pronation cascade. It is important to remember that tissue alignment does not necessarily imply force transfer between adjacent tissues, unless it has been proven.

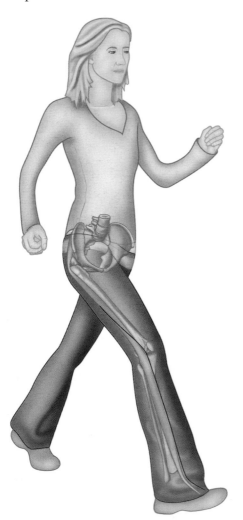

Figure 5.6. *If we follow the internal rotation forces through the lower limb at heel strike, we come to the hip extensor side of the "hip deltoid" and into the gluteus maximus, which will be firing to control hip adduction, flexion, and medial rotation.*

A lot of force is required to prevent the body from falling at heel strike, as the center of gravity is relatively far behind the point of support on the ground. Many muscles will be involved in counteracting the downward force, but the hip extensors, hip abductors, and biceps femoris have to contract particularly strongly (see fig. 5.7). The ability of these muscles to control the pronation cascade will be influenced by the amount of pre-tension they receive as a result of both stride length (chapter 3) and pelvic tilt (chapter 4). A reduced range of motion in these sagittal and frontal planes may reduce the potential force output of the gluteus maximus in particular, which has to work in all three planes.

The biceps femoris contracts with considerable force at heel strike (see fig. 5.7*A*). Thankfully, it is prepared for this by pre-tensioning prior to impact by the dorsiflexion of the foot. Toward the latter stages of the swing phase, the tibialis anterior draws the foot into dorsiflexion and some inversion, and this motion pulls on the fibularis longus, the tibialis anterior's antagonist in the dorsiflexion of the foot, but agonist in terms of force closing the foot's dome. This stretching of the fibularis longus brings the fibula downward and therefore lengthens the fascia of the biceps femoris (Vleeming et al. 2007). The biceps femoris is also stretched by the flexion of the hip. Being "separated" from both ends like this may help the biceps femoris fascia to increase the efficiency of the hip extensors' activation. Activating from inside this pre-tensioned fascial encasement, the biceps femoris contracts at heel strike with more efficiency.

Some of the force from the contraction of the biceps femoris may be transmitted into the fibularis longus, pulling the fibula upward again and tensioning the fibularis longus from above as the tibialis anterior relaxes. This action will assist the sequence of pronation events in the foot, since the fibularis longus helps

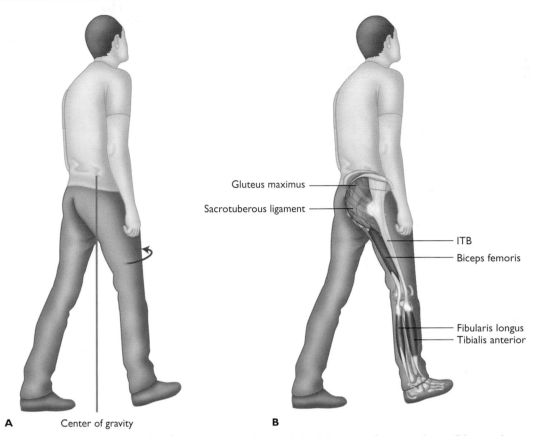

Gluteus maximus

Sacrotuberous ligament

ITB
Biceps femoris

Fibularis longus
Tibialis anterior

A Center of gravity   **B**

Figure 5.7.   A, In this position, with the hip flexed and the center of gravity behind the point of support, there will have to be a strong contraction within the hip extensors to prevent the body from falling. The biceps femoris is tensioned during the swing phase, prior to heel strike, by the hip flexion and by the supination of the foot, which tensions the myofascia of the fibularis longus. B, With eversion of the calcaneus and the chain of the medial rotations of the bones of the leg, there will be a consistent rotation from the hip to the sole of the foot.

to draw the midtarsal bones into eversion, which unlocks the joints, opening the foot and allowing it to adapt to the ground surface.

The use of the gluteus maximus and biceps femoris gives us control at heel strike on two separate myofascial levels. The deeper hamstrings will bring the force to the sacrum and sacroiliac joints (see "The Sacroiliac Joints" later in this chapter), and they will help decelerate knee flexion. The more superficial gluteus maximus connects to the opposite upper limb (see "Recruiting the Posterior Oblique Sling" below) and also links down through the ITB to the front of the knee to control against knee flexion and internal rotation.

After mid-stance, the TFL and the tibialis anterior are actively lengthened as the pelvis moves over the foot rockers and the hip extends. But, because of its more oblique fiber orientation, the TFL assists with rotation as well as hip flexion.

Deltoid of the Hip and Hydraulic Amplification

If we look at the lower limb following heel strike (see fig. 5.2), we can see a continual downward rotation pattern occurring as the foot pronates. This line of force connects the pronation of the foot to the lateral rotators of the hip, especially the upper portion of the gluteus maximus (see fig. 5.7B). The superior portion of the gluteus maximus and the tensor fasciae latae are encased within the same fascial layer and both will be contracting to stabilize the pelvis in the frontal plane (we saw earlier in chapters 1 and 4—see fig. 1.24).

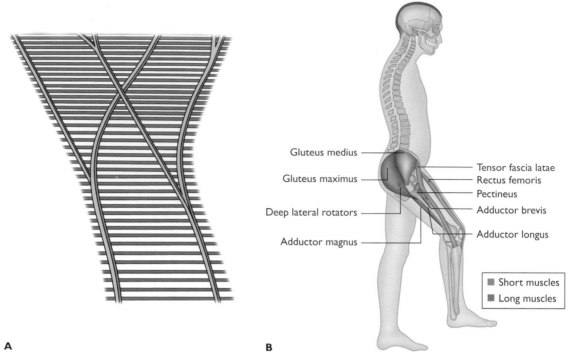

A   **B**

Figure 5.8.   *A,The greater trochanter is acting as what Myers calls a "switch" (or a "point" in the United Kingdom), the mechanism for changing tracks on a railway system. B,When the hip is flexed, the line of force travels posteriorly to the gluteus maximus; when extended, it goes to the tensor fasciae latae. The French anatomist Louis Hubert Farabeuf (1841–1910) suggested that the TFL/gluteus maximus/ITB should be considered a deltoid muscle and is sometimes referred to as the "deltoid of Farabeuf."*

The fascial sheets and the underlying muscle tissue can often cooperate to create a force amplification system called the *hydraulic amplifier effect*, as we saw in chapter 1 (see fig. 1.14*B*): tensioning the fascial sheets increases the efficiency of the associated muscles, either in series or in parallel. This can be brought about in a number of ways:

1. Tensioning of the muscles embedded within the sheet. This is seen with the tensor fasciae latae and the gluteus maximus (both of which are encased within the fascia lata), the platysma (within the fascia colli superficialis), and the pectoralis minor (contained within the clavipectoral fascia).
2. Contraction of muscles deep to the fascial layer. The contraction of the thigh muscles will tension the fascia lata from below, just as the erector spinae will tauten the posterior sheet of the thoracolumbar fascia.
3. Stretching and thereby elastically loading the tissue by the natural momentum of body movement. The swing of the arm will

tension the thoracolumbar fascia, while the swing of the leg will tension the epimysia of the hip extensors (fig. 5.8).

All three of these mechanisms can be, and often are, combined in real-life movement. It is estimated that the hydraulic amplifier can increase the efficiency of muscular work by up to 30 percent (DeRosa and Porterfield 2007), so it is clearly a mechanism that one would want to make full use of. When tensioning of the fascial sheets is disrupted, such as by a fasciotomy, approximately 12 to 16 percent of efficiency can be lost (Gracovetsky 2008).

As the pelvis moves over the planted foot, the line of force will move from the gluteus maximus to the tensor fasciae latae, or from the extensor to the flexor (see fig. 5.2; this was also explored in chapter 3—Sagittal Plane), bringing us to the front of the hip again. In chapter 4 we saw that the deltoid of Farabeuf is tensioned throughout the stance period, as it controls flexion/extension, adduction, and medial rotation of the hip. The tensional relationship of this muscular deltoid with the fascia lata therefore assists the muscles of the thigh by providing a taut superficial bag for them to work within.

The relationship between contraction of the gluteus maximus at heel strike and control of the knee is well established, and failure to slow the internal rotation and frontal plane motion of the joint is often related to overpronation of the foot or to muscle weakness (Ireland et al. 2003; Powers et al. 2003). The relationship of the hip joint to the inside of the foot is therefore well documented, and the line of force can be clearly observed—especially when it is exaggerated, such as in landing after a jump or changing direction while running.

It is important enough to reiterate that a weak gluteus maximus is often blamed when the pronation cascade appears uncontrolled, but this is not necessarily the case. We regularly pre-tension the myofascia by lengthening it in two planes and then have to control the movement in the third; if insufficient loading occurs in one of the other planes, we lose the advantage for decelerating the third. Therefore, when looking at a possibly weak gluteus maximus, we need to check if the hip is adducting enough (to strain it frontally) and flexing enough (to strain it sagittally) so that it needs less concentric contraction to control the transverse lengthening.

Recruiting the Posterior Oblique Sling—Connecting the Upper to the Lower Limb

The gluteus maximus is also strongly connected to the latissimus dorsi on the opposite side of the body, and this relationship is renowned for its ability to increase stability. This connection has been thoroughly investigated by Vleeming (posterior sling) and Zorn ("swingwalker"), as well as by Myers (Back Functional Line). Vleeming and Zorn both used the well-supported contralateral connections from the latissimus dorsi to the upper gluteus maximus, while Myers chose to use the latissimus dorsi connection to the opposite vastus lateralis via the lower portion of the gluteus maximus, even though this connection is considered quite variable (Wilke et al. 2016). Whichever functional sling one chooses, they each connect from the outside of the knee at heel strike (ITB for Vleeming, or vastus lateralis for Myers) all the way to the opposite humerus (latissimus dorsi), both of which should be traveling in opposing directions on the transverse plane. The knee will be coming across into a valgus position, while the opposite arm is swinging forward and into a little external rotation, distally tensioning both ends of the obliquely oriented line of tissue. The movement of the contralateral limb bones creates a long diagonal sling passing around the back of the flexed hip (via the thoracolumbar fascia, with the gluteus maximus and latissimus dorsi attaching to it), which can then catapult the pelvis forward (see fig. 5.9A, and, for more information on the role of the thoracolumbar fascia/gluteus maximus link for energy saving, visit Adjo Zorn's site: www.swingwalker.net).

Once the pelvis has moved in front of the supporting foot, the line of force then engages through the tensor fasciae latae (although it is a medial rotator of the thigh, it will be stretched and opened by the hip extension), and, through the potential continuity of the tibialis anterior, it may help lift the medial arch and will bring the femur, tibia, and fibula, as well as the first metatarsal, into a lateral rotation (see fig. 5.10).

Exercise 5.1. **You can feel the relationship between the feet and the pelvis when standing comfortably with feet approximately hip-width apart and slowly tilting the pelvis anteriorly and posteriorly. In an anterior tilt, you may feel the knees overextend as the bones medially rotate and the medial arches of the foot lower. With a posterior tilt, you should feel the knees soften and the bones laterally rotate as the medial arches lift.**

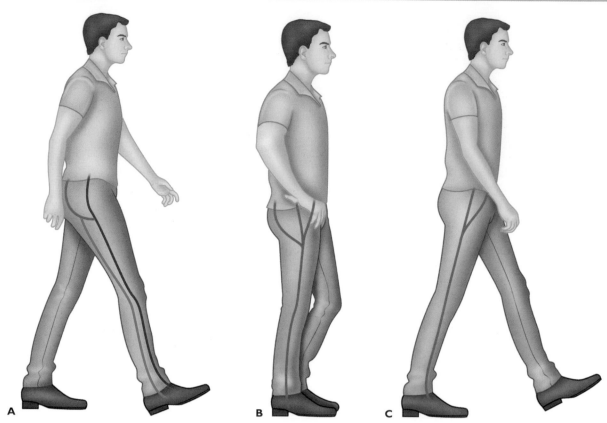

Figure 5.9. *At the point of contact, there has to be a strong contraction in the extensors as well as the abductors. The extensors are pre-stretched by the hip flexion, and the abductors by the lateral shift of the pelvis creating adduction of the hip, as we saw in chapter 4. The opposite shoulder girdle adds support to the extended lower limb via the latissimus dorsi to the supporting gluteus maximus and down the front of the leg with the ITB and tibialis anterior. The gluteus maximus is therefore being pre-stretched by opposite shoulder movement as well as by the hip flexion and adduction. All of this increases the body's potential efficiency through elastic recoil. As the pelvis moves over the planted foot, the line of force from the body's center of gravity moves from behind (A) to in line (B) and finally in front (C) of the point of support. This moves the need for contraction through the so-called "deltoid of the hip" (gluteus maximus, gluteus medius, and tensor fasciae latae).*

EMG, Mechanoreceptors, and Movement

By using the overlay of EMG readings alongside the gait cycle, we can see how muscles respond to movement. For example, the EMG readings for the hip extensors show that most of these muscles begin to contract prior to heel strike. The biceps femoris and semimembranosus start to contract as early as mid-swing (see fig. 5.11); the adductor magnus, gluteus maximus, and gluteus medius also begin to fire before contact is made with the ground. These early contractions are best explained by the need to slow the forward swing of the leg. They serve to prepare the fascial tissue for the loading at heel strike, once again increasing the efficiency of muscular contractions through pre-tension of the myofascial tissue.

It seems logical that the preparatory contraction is initiated by the straining of the fascia as the thigh comes forward into hip flexion. The strain within the fascial tissue stimulates the appropriate mechanoreceptors to create tone in the extensors in preparation for the immediate absorption of the natural "give" in the tissue around the joints, negating the need to quickly decelerate the movement, as would be necessary if the muscles were totally quiescent on landing.

After heel strike, the anterior compartment rapidly lengthens because of the eversion and plantar flexion of the foot, and, remembering the work of Huijing (discussed in chapter 1), we can imagine the dispersal of mechanical information that will happen in response to this (see fig. 5.12). If this type of movement in the tissue is monitored by the mechanoreceptors

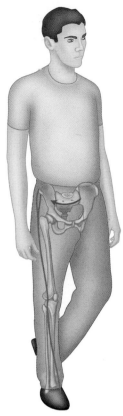

Figure 5.10. *Once the pelvis moves in front of the foot, the hip is in extension and therefore begins to lengthen the tensor fasciae latae. This engagement allows the anterior tissues to assist with the lift of the medial longitudinal arch, and the medial rotation of the hip will pull on the lateral rotators to encourage the femur and tibia to laterally rotate to help reengage the midtarsal joints.*

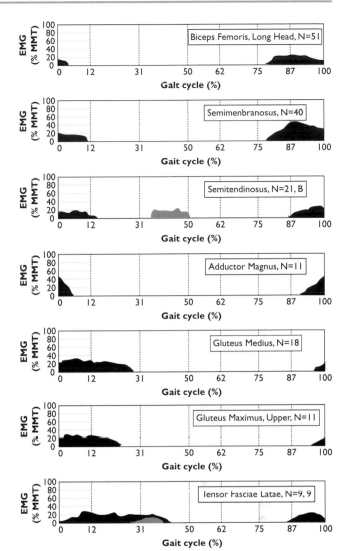

Figure 5.11. *EMG charts showing percentage of maximum manual muscle test (MMT) and the phase of gait at which each muscle is active. We can clearly see that the hip extensors are firing before they are required to accept the weight of the body, from mid-swing to late swing (75–100%), and then following through to give their support in heel strike (0–2%) and into mid-stance (12–31%). (Adapted from Perry and Burnfield 2010.)*

(and research suggests that it is), it again seems reasonable to assume that changes in fascial tension are at least partially responsible for the stimulation of local muscle fibers.

Movement of the fascia helps activate the appropriate muscles for the control of each phase, and the muscles should switch on naturally and reflexively. During the mid- to late swing phase, it is the posterior hip extensors that are turned on, and then, once the foot is planted and the limb begins to rotate, the transverse plane vector will further stimulate the gluteus maximus as well as the tibialis anterior. In both cases, the muscles are activated by the lengthening of their myofascia. The momentum of the leg swing stimulates the hip extensors, and the rotation of the bones following the initial contact with the ground turns on the tibialis anterior and gluteus maximus.

The EMG readings for the anterior tissues show an alternation between the active portions of the gait cycle, during which force must be carried or absorbed and work is performed by the muscle tissue to resist ground reaction force or build momentum, and a more passive phase of the gait cycle, during which the correction of position or initiation of an action is made by the fibrous elements, preferably through elastic energy. Both the swing phase of the thigh and the correction of the medial longitudinal arch occur when the tensor fasciae latae and the tibialis anterior are electrically quiet, indicating a greater possibility of fascial involvement (see fig. 5.13).

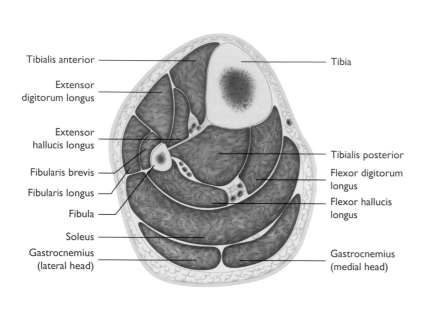

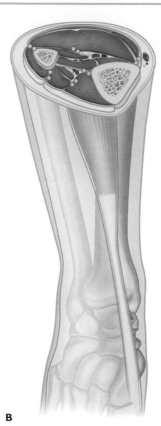

Tibialis anterior — Tibia
Extensor digitorum longus
Extensor hallucis longus
Fibularis brevis — Tibialis posterior
Fibularis longus — Flexor digitorum longus
Fibula — Flexor hallucis longus
Soleus
Gastrocnemius (lateral head) — Gastrocnemius (medial head)

A

B

Figure 5.12. A, A change in tension, due to the ground reaction force and the downward pull of gravity, will send the force of the adjustment into the surrounding tissue, not just into the tibialis anterior. Presumably the tissue will be receiving signals from many other sources and then, on recognizing patterns, can create the necessary response in the muscle tone. B, Many mechanoreceptors are located in or around the septal divisions, which are the main borders between the muscles. The mechanoreceptors sense the variations in tension and shearing forces. Essentially, these areas are experiencing the most relative change, and so it makes sense to place the mechanoreceptors along these interfaces.

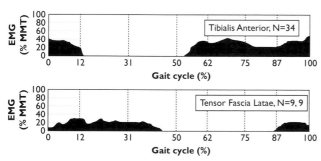

Figure 5.13. The EMG readings show the tibialis anterior as being electrically active from pre-swing (53%) through to mid-stance (12%). Presumably, it is stimulated during the swing phase by the weight of the foot loading the fascial tissue. The mechanoreceptors are stimulated and signal the muscle to lift the foot during the swing—to keep it clear of the ground—and then the muscle is quickly unloaded after receiving the forces of body weight and momentum. The tensor fasciae latae, as an abductor, is active through almost all of the stance phase, but it trails off before the leg swing occurs. This appears to indicate a passive mechanism for the hip flexion, as would be suggested by its recoil ability (and as felt in exercise 3.1). (Adapted from Perry and Burnfield 2010.)

Pelvic and Thoracic Rotation—Ipsilateral

I set off. What a gait. Stiffness of the lower limbs, as if nature had denied me knees, extraordinary splaying of the feet to the right and left of the line of march. The trunk, on the contrary, as if by the effect of a compensatory mechanism, was as flabby as an old ragbag, tossing wildly to the unpredictable jolts of the pelvis.

—Samuel Beckett, *First Love and Other Novellas*

Provided we can turn the pelvis during gait and, unlike Beckett's walker above, have

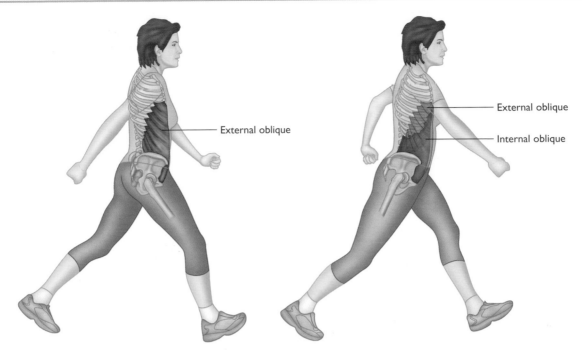

External oblique

External oblique

Internal oblique

Figure 5.14. *At full stride, there is a relative rotation between the pelvis and the thorax, which is controlled (and also limited!) by the alternate obliques on either side. This arrangement allows the body to be stable in both the frontal and transverse planes by contracting different proportions of the internal and external obliques on both sides.*

enough strength to control it, a rotation should carry up the body as well as down the legs. The rotation travels through the waist, the abdominals, and the intercostals in a series of crossed tissues (see fig. 5.14), which makes sense when viewing the contralateral positions achieved at heel strike and toe-off. When the feet are at heel strike and toe-off, the pelvis will be rotated toward the side of the extended leg, as described in chapter 3. This creates a relative rotation between the pelvis and the thorax, and so the direction of force required for stability between the pelvis and the rib cage will not be vertical but will be at an oblique angle (see fig. 5.14). The oblique tissues therefore play a role in supporting the ilium on the toe-off/ swing side.

The oblique muscles also affect, and are affected by, the length of stride, either decelerating or limiting the amount of rotation between the thorax and the pelvis as we reach full stride length. Therefore, if a client shows the thorax and pelvis rotating at the same or a similar rate—or if one shows a limited

stride length (which would serve to minimize rotation)—the range of motion of the obliques should be examined.

The rotation between the pelvis and the rib cage allows the intercostals to also contribute their energy to gait. For this to occur, there must be enough movement between the pelvis and the rib cage to stretch and engage the thoracic musculature. Movement between the pelvis and the thorax will require not only the spinal involvement described below but also the opposite-side internal and external obliques to be long enough and strong enough to carry the forces.

The ipsilateral oblique tissues can be easily tested by having the client rotate his or her rib cage or lunge forward to assess the amount of available movement. Palpating the area as the client performs the test can give the necessary feedback, as the therapist will be able to feel if the obliques limit the movement or if they remain loose and uninvolved (see fig. 5.15).

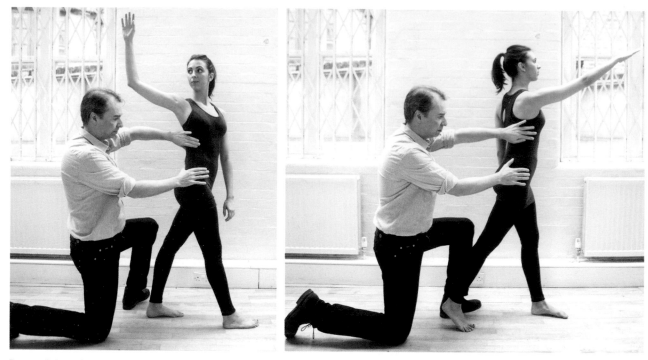

Figure 5.15.   *By palpating the muscles of the waist on both sides, the therapist can assess the range of motion of the obliques and the amount of strength available from them. Thoracic rotation and anterior lunging can be used while the therapist feels for any variation in quality between the external obliques on one side and the internal obliques on the other.*

Pelvic, Thoracic, and Shoulder Rotation—Contralateral

The rib cage and ilia are connected on the same side by the lateral obliques, and we can also follow the diagonal line to the opposite-side rib cage, which leads into the upper attachments of the external obliques. These attachments are superficial to the myofascial level of the intercostals, which are deeper in the body and follow the "core", or the torso; instead, the obliques will lead us to the shoulder girdles via the serratus anterior.

Although the tissue of the tensor fasciae latae has not been shown to continue into that of the internal oblique (Wilke et al. 2016), the line of force created during the gait cycle is continuous and travels up away from the anterior superior iliac spine (ASIS). The continuity of the direction of force takes us across the abdomen from the internal obliques to the opposite external obliques. From the external obliques, the line of force continues with the serratus anterior, and there have been a number of studies that do report myofascial continuity between these three tissues (Wilke et al. 2016; Stecco and Hammer 2015).

The difference between the ipsilateral and contralateral obliques is that the former takes the rotation into the pliable rib cage, while the latter utilizes the opposite shoulder girdle, and thereby brings the arm movement and momentum into the equation for the counterrotation.

The organization of the obliques and serratus anterior takes the tissue from being anchored on the trunk to being part of the shoulder girdle. The myofascial line then returns to the trunk at the spinous processes to meet the splenius capitis and cervicis. This change in depth allows the shoulder girdles and the trunk to rotate independently of each other, contributing to our contralateral arm/leg swing; we can see this arrangement when we look at the body from the top (see fig. 5.16).

Thus, the tissue organization of the trunk gives us three layers of rotation. The deepest is the

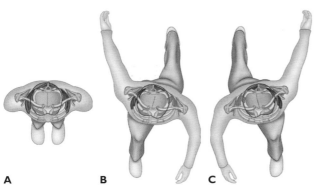

A   **B**   **C**

Figure 5.16. The oblique tissues of the upper body give us an axial-to-appendicular-to-axial link in the skeleton (A), which allows one to rotate independently of the other (B). However, this portion of myofascial tissue cannot be consistently short or long through its entirety: when the portion inferior to the medial border of the scapula is short (B), the superior portion will be long, and vice versa (C).

rotation of the spine created by the turning of the pelvis and therefore the sacrum. A middle layer of force is carried by the ipsilateral obliques to the rib cage and intercostals. The most superficial—and the counterrotation to the others—is carried via the contralateral obliques, serratus anterior, rhomboids, and opposite splenii. This counterrotation creates an external "balance spring" to the others. During relaxed walking, it seems to help dissipate the rotational forces prior to reaching the head, while during vigorous walking, it is more actively engaged (whether held more stiffly or through concentric/eccentric contraction) and contributes a stronger counterrotation (see also "The Spinal Engine" later in this chapter).

Our arm swing is contralateral to the swing of the lower limb—when one arm is back, the leg on the opposite side will also be back. As we saw above, the hip flexors (including the tensor fasciae latae) passively assists the leg swing through fascial recoil. The leg swing may also be assisted by the oblique tissues of the upper body, because of the shoulder being back and the pelvis dropping and rotating away from the rib cage on the opposite side (see fig. 5.17); this creates an aligned series of tissues to act as an anchor for the transverse plane force created by the pelvic rotation.

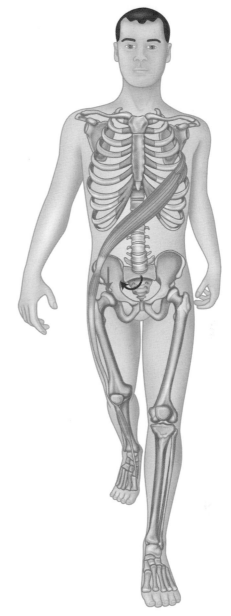

Figure 5.17. As the arm swings back, it helps to fascially engage the anterior Spiral Line from the medial border of one scapula to the opposite first metatarsal. The tension of the myofascia of the oblique tissues is enhanced by the pelvis shifting to the opposite side, adducting and rotating. Each of these movements increases the distance from the scapula to the opposite anterior superior iliac spine. We will see this contralateral pattern again later, as part of the Anterior Oblique Sling.

In the extended position prior to toe-off (fig. 5.17), we see a continuous line of force that matches Myers proposed Spiral Line. However, the fascial continuity between the internal oblique and the TFL has been questioned (Wilke et al. 2016). As we saw with the obliques and abductors in the frontal plane, a lack of fascial connection between the two muscles would make sense from a functional point of view, as the pelvis requires stability from above, while the TFL assists with the imminent hip flexion. Force communication between these two muscles at this phase could decrease stability, whereas controlling the pelvis on either side of the ASIS anchors the pelvis between the opposing forces.

As we see in fig. 5.16, when the right leg is extended, the pelvis—and therefore the spinal vertebrae—rotate to the right. The shoulder girdle will be forward on the right, and if we look at the obliquely oriented posterior tissues (see fig. 5.17), we can clearly see that the

forward momentum of the right shoulder creates a stretch on the spinous processes of the mid- and upper thoracic spine. This may help produce the counterrotation of the spine, or at least reduce the rotation created by the pelvis before it reaches the head.

There is an alternating pattern of stretch in the upper oblique tissues: as the tissue on the front of the trunk is stretched on one side by the posterior swing of the arm, the tissue on the back of the other side is shortened (see figs. 5.17 and 5.18). This is allowed by the paradoxical relationship of the rhomboid-serratus sling, the two sides of which cannot be short (or long) at the same time.

■ THE SACROILIAC JOINTS

Stride length appears to influence the sacroiliac joint (SIJ) and the three-dimensional movement through the pelvic complex in healthy walking. When the left and right feet are at the extremes of the gait cycle—heel strike and toe-off— the corresponding ilium will be relatively posteriorly and anteriorly tilted, respectively (see fig. 5.19), creating a torsion through the pelvis. If we heel strike with the right foot, the right ilium will be posteriorly tilted (you can feel this on yourself if you are not familiar with it). The ilium moves further and faster than the sacrum, so the sacrum will be anteriorly tilted relative to the ilium on the right side. This relationship is known as *nutation* (see fig. 5.19).

As we heel strike on the right, we will be preparing for toe-off on the left, and this will create the opposite tilts of the ilium and sacrum on the left side, thereby causing a relative posterior tilt, or *counter-nutation*, of the sacrum at the left sacroiliac joint.[1]

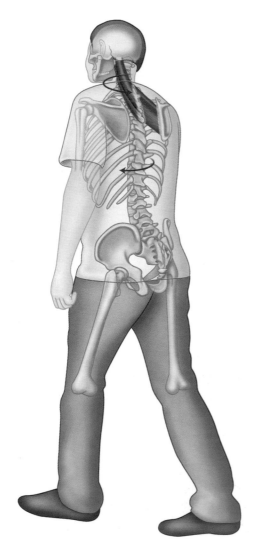

Figure 5.18.   *As the arm swings forward, it creates a pull through the rhomboids and the splenii, which may help reduce the spinal rotation coming from the pelvis.*

[1]The use of "counter-nutation" at the sacroiliac joint in function is debated, as some argue that the sacroiliac joints are always nutated in weight bearing. I use it here to describe the joint's position relative to the opposite side, not the actual position at the joint.

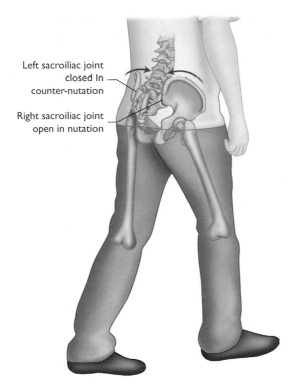

Left sacroiliac joint closed In counter-nutation

Right sacroiliac joint open in nutation

Figure 5.19. When the heel strikes, the femur will be posteriorly tilted, drawing the ilium with it, while the reverse relationship will be occurring on the opposite side. This creates a nutation on the side of heel strike and a counter-nutation on the other.

The torsional nutation and counter-nutation through the pelvis are corrected naturally through the mechanics of weight acceptance, stance, and swing phase.

The sacrum sits in the pelvis like a hammock, with the dorsal sacroiliac ligaments supporting it like ropes from the trees of the ilia (see fig. 5.20A). The anterior tilt of the human pelvis is in contrast to the ape's, whose pelvis sits almost parallel to the spine. The evolution of the human pelvis appears to provide the sacroiliac joints with the ability to reduce the forces coming from the lower limbs before these forces reach the spine. The suspension arrangement of the sacroiliac joints and their nutation/counter-nutation movements create a natural shock absorber that tolerates relative motion in all three planes of movement.

Restriction in the sacroiliac joints transfers more movement from the ilia to the sacrum and spine. If the ligaments are unable to allow movement, the sacrum will be forced to follow

the movement of the ilia, and then the L5 vertebra will be forced to follow the sacrum. The client, however, may compensate with less lower limb movement, especially limiting their hip flexion and extension, to reduce the tilting of the ilia.

Although the nutation and counter-nutation movements of the pelvis are very small, they must be contained. Control of this movement is one of many functions of the sacroiliac ligaments and may be assisted by their continuity with contractile tissues on either side of the sacroiliac complex. A number of reports demonstrate a variable continuity between the biceps femoris and the sacrotuberous ligament; however, van Wingerden et al. (1993) showed that force can be transferred between these structures regardless of the amount of fascial continuity. Tensioning of the surrounding ligaments is part of the force-closure mechanism for support of the sacroiliac joints; this tension comes both from the ligaments' passive reaction to the wind-up created by the torsion through the pelvis, and from their continuity with contractile tissues (Vleeming et al. 2012).

Jap van Der Waal, a Dutch anatomist, recently revisited work from his 1988 doctoral thesis which developed the concept of "dynaments" (his suggested contraction of "dynamic ligament"). In his model, based on many dissections, he suggests that we should reconsider the idea that ligaments are primarily passive supporting structures. Instead, he shows that most ligaments actually lie in series with the contractile tissue (i.e., they are continuous with the muscle) and are therefore tensioned by it. In this case, we should consider the sacrotuberous ligament as an extended tendon of the hamstrings— of the biceps femoris in particular (Willard, in Vleeming et al. 2007). The implication of this is that the sacrotuberous ligament has an active functional role—it encourages the return of the sacrum from a nutated position

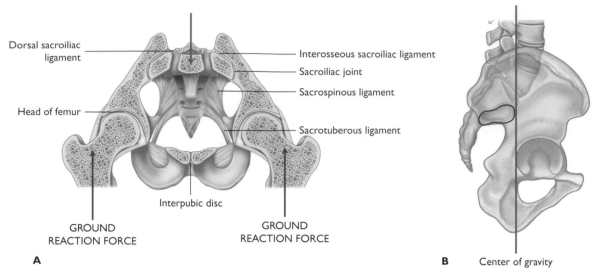

Dorsal sacroiliac ligament

Interosseous sacroiliac ligament

Sacroiliac joint

Sacrospinous ligament

Head of femur

Sacrotuberous ligament

Interpubic disc

GROUND REACTION FORCE

GROUND REACTION FORCE

A

B   Center of gravity

Figure 5.20.   From the cross section in the frontal plane (A), we can see how the sacrum is suspended from the ilia. This arrangement allows each of the three bones to move relative to the others. If we imagine the sacrum in the middle as a hammock and the dorsal sacroiliac ligaments as the ropes, the ilia are therefore like the supporting trees. B, The arrangement is enhanced by the almost horizontal orientation of the sacrum, which increases slightly when in standing (SIJ outlined in purple).

(see fig. 5.21). This is a reversal of roles: the passive job of the ligaments (the prevention of movement) is altered by the incorporation of an active contraction, making them an "in-series" extension of the muscular elements and thereby involved in the creation of movement.

On the opposite side of the sacrum, the long dorsal sacroiliac ligament "officially" helps prevent counter-nutation. This ligament is connected to the erector spinae and to some extent to the multifidi. Vleeming and Stoeckart found that tractioning the erectors led to an increase in tension in the long dorsal sacroiliac ligament (in Vleeming et al. 2007). We can see how this ligament can behave as a "dynament" and create nutation on contraction of the lower back extensors.

Follow the exercise below and you will feel a contralateral relationship between the hamstrings and the erectors at the point of heel strike (the multifidi and the erectors will activate on both sides of the spine but more so on the "swing side"). By following the tissue to the opposite side of the sacrum via this functional sling of sacrotuberous to long dorsal

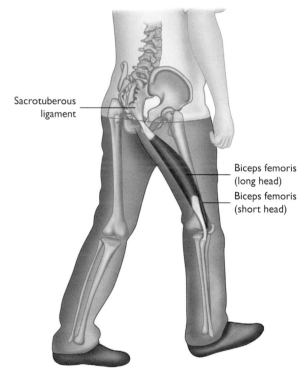

Sacrotuberous ligament

Biceps femoris (long head)

Biceps femoris (short head)

Figure 5.21.   The contraction of the biceps femoris on heel strike and the loading to prevent further hip flexion creates tension that must be carried through onto the sacrotuberous ligament. This contraction prevents additional nutation of the sacroiliac joint and may also help its return to a neutral position.

sacroiliac ligament, we now have an oblique tensioning of support and correction for the action of the SIJs (see fig. 5.21).

Exercise 5.2. **Place your right hand on your right hamstrings and the back of your left hand across the erector spinae of your lower back and take a few steps. What do you feel at the point of heel strike on the right?**

Hopefully you feel a strong tensioning of the hamstrings on the right and of the erector spinae on the left (see figs. 5.21 to 5.23).

Repeat exercise 3.3 to feel the opposing motions of the ilia in walking (the ilium on the side of heel strike should be tilting back). Imagine what is happening to the sacroiliac joint inside. As the ilium tilts back, it moves further than the sacrum, making it "nutate" relative to the position of the sacrum.

Feel—and then picture—what is happening on the extended limb: the ilium is anteriorly

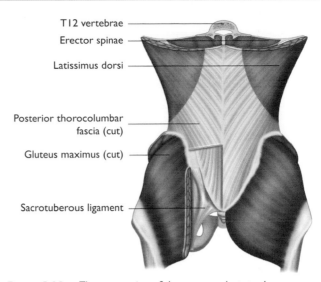

Figure 5.23. *The contraction of the erectors deep to the tensioned thoracolumbar fascia will also assist with the "hydraulic amplification" in this segment.*

tilting and the sacroiliac joint is counter-nutating. Imagine a line between the sacrotuberous ligament and the posterior superior iliac spine and feel this as the axis of correction. As you step, can you internally sense that line becoming taut to help correct the torsion that occurs in the sacroiliac joint?

■ DEEP LONGITUDINAL SLING

In the first edition of this book I explored Myers' Spiral Line and made some changes to Myers' original outline contained in the first and second editions of *Anatomy Trains* (2001, 2009). My discoveries were then incorporated by Myers for his third edition of *Anatomy Trains* (2015; see fig. 5.24), showing a switch from the biceps femoris and sacrotuberous ligament on one side to the long dorsal sacroiliac ligament and erector spinae on the opposite side. At the time of writing, I was unaware that this continuity had already been suggested by Vleeming and formed what he calls the *Deep Longitudinal Sling*. As Vleeming's work predates my own, my preference is therefore to present in this edition his idea of the functional and myofascial continuity.

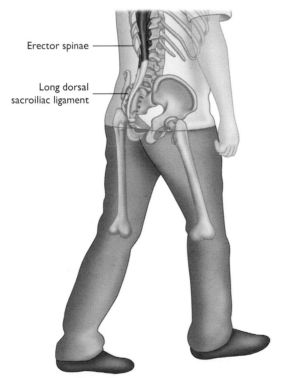

Figure 5.22. *With the long dorsal sacroiliac ligament now in place, you can see the axis that may help with the three-dimensional movement of the sacrum in the sacroiliac joint.*

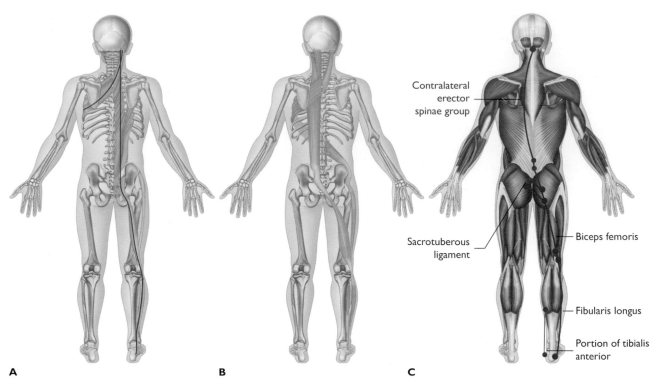

A   **B**   **C**

Figure 5.24.   *A, Myers' original Spiral Line ascended the back of the body along the same side from foot to head (Myers 2001 and 2009). B, Following suggestions based on functional rather than structural relationships, Myers changed the Spiral Line to swap sides at the sacrum (Myers 2015). C, Vleeming's Deep Longitudinal Sling includes the tibialis anterior, fibularis longus, biceps femoris, sacrotuberous and dorsal sacroiliac ligaments, and erector spinae.*

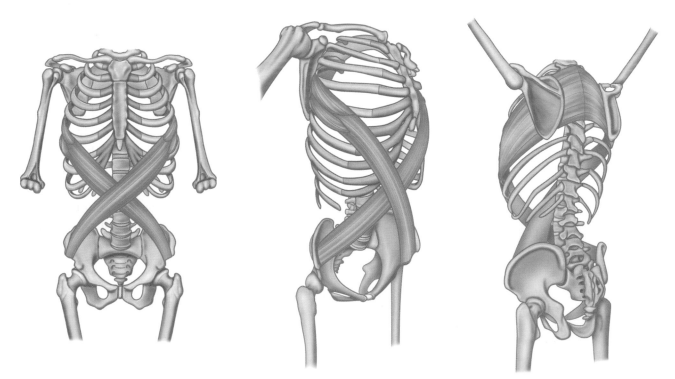

Figure 5.25.   *This image shows the spiral relationship through the torso, from one anterior superior iliac spine through the shoulder girdles to the opposite anterior superior iliac spine. This is in contrast to Myers's Spiral Line, which includes the lower limbs and assists with the body's rotational patterns.*

■ THE SPINAL ENGINE

One does not need legs to be a nomad.

—Zygmunt Bauman

The body has many obliquely oriented tissues (figs. 5.24 & 5.25) to facilitate contralateral movement during gait. Gracovetsky posits, in his Spinal Engine Theory, that the three sections of the spine function cooperatively during the rotations of walking (see fig. 5.26). The pelvis and lumbars are coupled together in rotation, as discussed earlier in chapter 3 (see also fig. 5.26): when the lower limbs are in flexion and extension, the pelvis rotates to accommodate the length of the stride. The inability of the lumbars to absorb all of the rotation (because of their limitations in the transverse plane; see fig. 5.27) sends the rotational forces up to the thoracics, which, as a result of the counterrotation of the shoulder girdles, creates fascial tensioning and wind-up in the rotatores and multifidi. According to Gracovetsky, these two rotations should ideally meet somewhere around T8 and act somewhat like a watch spring. The natural momentum of the rotation serves to tension the tissues, which then recoil into the reverse rotation. Using spinal facet and oblique tissue alignment, Gracovetsky argues that we do not require the lower limbs for movement—the two rotations from the upper body are enough to propel us forward.

The forward swing of the arm tensions the rhomboids and opposite-side splenii, which helps to rotate the upper thoracic spine and the head in the opposite direction to that of the lumbars and lower thoracics. This counterrotation of the spine and rib cage neutralizes the rotation of the lower body, helping to stabilize the head in the transverse plane.

The oblique "dynaments" of Vleeming's Deep Posterior Sling therefore add a mechanism to correct the torsion of the pelvis via the two sacral ligaments, as well as helping to create Gracovetsky's "Spinal Engine" mechanism.

The ipsilateral obliques bring the rotation of the pelvis into the rib cage, and then the more superficial serape effect of the rhomboids and serratus anterior uses the counterrotation of the shoulders to add opposing transverse forces into the equation, producing greater efficiency for the transverse plane movement and taking advantage of the spinal mechanics.

Obliquely oriented tissues are involved in nearly all the movements necessary for walking—foot pronation and its correction to supination, the rotations and flexions and extensions of the lower limbs, the movement at the sacrum and into the spine, and the rotation of the trunk and counterrotations of the shoulder girdles—all of which help to keep the head steady.

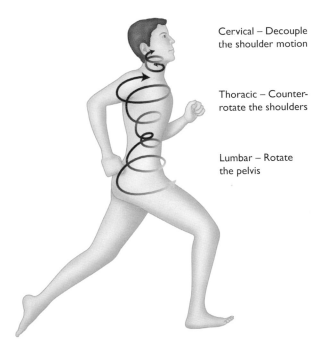

Cervical – Decouple the shoulder motion

Thoracic – Counter-rotate the shoulders

Lumbar – Rotate the pelvis

Figure 5.26. *The three spinal sections, according to Gracovetsky, contribute to the transverse motion of gait. The lumbars move with the pelvis, and the thoracics counterrotate because of the shoulder girdle, leading to tensioning in the oblique muscles of the spine. The cervical region is uncoupled from the rest of the spine, both in its facet arrangement and through the arrangement of the soft tissue, which allows it to maintain the forward gaze of the head. (Adapted from Gracovetsky 2008.)*

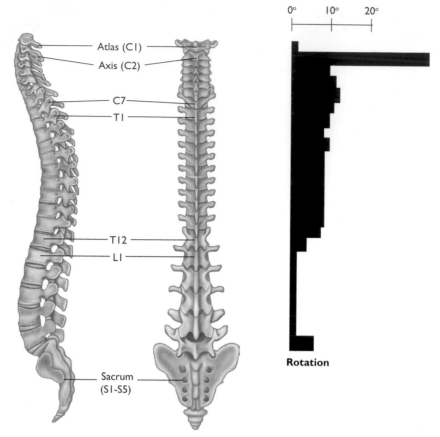

Figure 5.27. *Because of limited rotation in the lumbars, their ability to absorb transverse plane movement is reduced. The pelvic rotation caused by the reach of the forward leg therefore transfers into the thoracic vertebrae, as described in chapter 4, as it is carried upward via the "X" of the obliques. The facets of the thoracic vertebrae are aligned a little more in the frontal plane and thereby allow more rotation. The counterrotation of the upper girdle then encourages a meeting of these opposing rotations around the level of T8, producing a fascial recoil in the transverse plane. Note that this is a simplified non-functional view of spinal movement—the actual ranges will change once the spine moves from neutral. (Adapted from Middleditch and Oliver 2005.)*

■ ESSENTIAL EVENTS

Pronation/Supination

The talar joint allows sagittal plane movements, while the subtalar (talocalcaneal joint) enables inversion and eversion. We have to put them in context with the even-longer-named talocalcaneonavicular joint (a rounded ball-and-socket type joint) and the calcaneocuboid joint (a gliding joint). It is the latter two joints that allow the movements of supination and pronation, which lock and unlock the midtarsal joints, respectively.

The fact that transverse plane movement is limited in the talar joint means that the rotation of the talus bone is coupled into the lower limb to create a series of medial rotations following heel strike. Stability is then returned to the foot via lateral rotation of the femur, tibia, and fibula from mid-stance to toe-off and is driven by the swing of the opposite leg. The lateral rotation of the bones will then couple across the talar joint to help correct the foot by creating "form" closure. However, the amount of lateral rotation will be related to the length of the stride, which could be affected by all of the sagittal plane essential events. These sagittal plane essential events could be counteracted by adding more rotation into the system in a compensated pattern.

The bones of the client's feet should be able to open and adapt on heel strike and then reengage in preparation for toe-off. This can be assessed to some degree during gait, but it will be easier to see by having the client move his or her knee over the medial and lateral aspects of the foot. These actions will create internal and external rotation of the talus, causing the foot to pronate and supinate (see fig. 5.28). First, do the test in a relaxed standing position, moving one leg at a time; this removes any other possible restrictions that may interfere with the test.

In the second stage of the test, the client stands in a more gait-like position to mimic the tissue relationships of walking (see fig. 5.29).

Sacroiliac Joint Mobility

For the pelvis to torsion correctly, with the ilia traveling in opposite directions, the sacroiliac joints must be mobile. A restriction on one side could lead to overextension on the other, as well as uneven loading into the spine.

There are many tests to assess the sacroiliac joints and they often give contradictory results. The therapist can assess the joints in the context of a normal gait, by feeling for the torsion as the

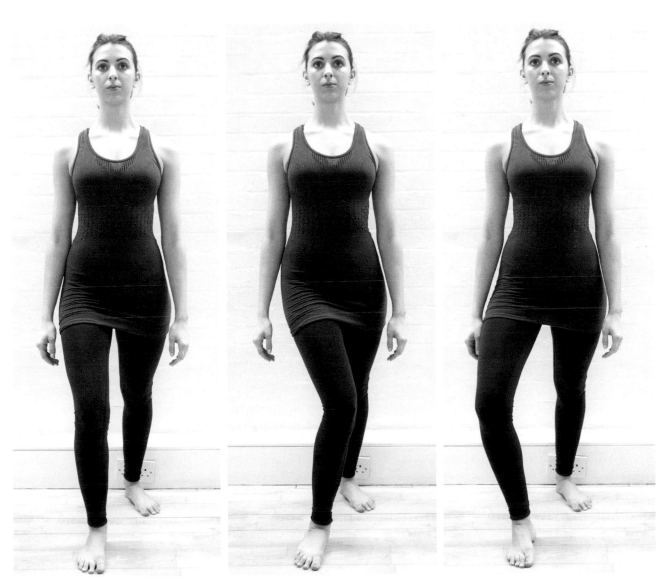

Figure 5.28. *In this first position, the client is relaxed and simply moves the knee medially and laterally, which should create pronation and supination, respectively. To assess this ability in gait see fig 5.29*

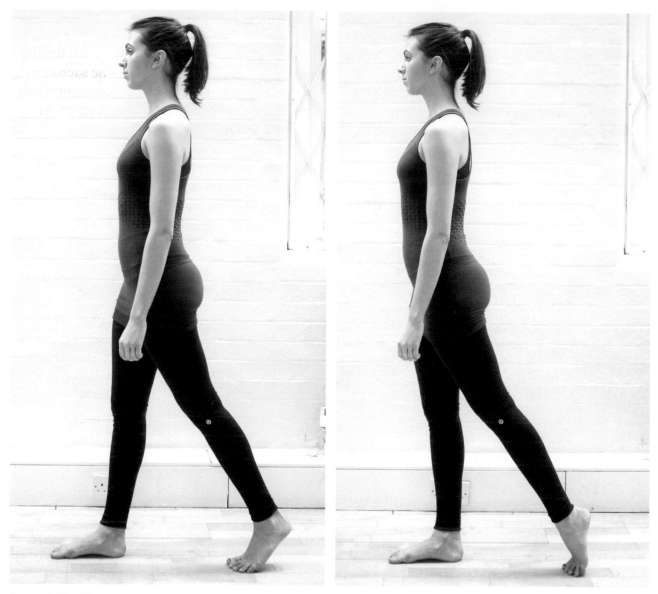

Figure 5.29.   Using a split stance, transfer the body weight onto the forward foot to assess for pronation of the front foot.

client either walks or transfers his or her body weight forward and back while standing in a position similar to that used in fig. 5.29.

Shoulder Girdle Counter-Swing

Various studies have shown that the arm swing adds little to the efficiency of gait. This seems to be a case of "science" saying one thing and experience saying another. The quote of Nicholson which helps open chapter 1 ("Walking while nursing an injured arm in a cast throws off your balance and distorts your geometry of the walking body, creating various tensions and asymmetries that in themselves create further pain") attests to the idea that— while not essential to walking—our arms do add a certain *je ne sais quoi*. Try walking at speed without swinging your arms, and you will feel their loss—or, as Nicholson did, try walking with one arm in a heavy cast.

Imbalances in arm swing can be clues to further weaknesses in the system. Too much swing, especially on one side, can indicate weak gluteal muscles, as the latissimus dorsi tries to compensate through the Posterior Oblique Sling (latissimus dorsi to opposite gluteus maximus and ITB). Insufficient swing (or lack of swing) may be due to shortness in this sling: a short Posterior Oblique Sling and a longer arm swing could encourage too much rotation of the opposite femur.

An overall increase in swing can indicate a lack of rotation through the thoracic cage, because increased swing can compensate for such immobility.

Arm swing can be dependent on the speed of movement, so assessing the client at varying speeds can be useful. With increased speed, expect an increased range of arm swing.

Thoracic Rotation

The forward step of the leg rotates the pelvis to one side, while both shoulder girdles lag behind in opposition and create a rotational counterbalance. The thorax twists as it is held between these two counterrotatory forces, and, provided the vertebral and costal joints have the relevant freedom of movement, the obliquely oriented tissues of the intercostals, spinal multifidi, and rotatores will be tensioned along with the abdominal obliques.

For the thorax to rotate, the shoulder girdles need to counter the rotation of the pelvis, and, if the pelvis tilts, coupled motion is sent up the spine in the form of both rotation and side flexion to engage the deep spinal muscles.

■ SUMMARY

1. Rotation is created through the body by a series of offset forces. The momentum of one leg swinging forward as the other remains planted causes the pelvis to turn between them. The offset between gravity and mass coming onto the sustentaculum tali and the ground reaction force coming up from the calcaneal tuberosity causes the talus to turn.
2. Pre-tension in the hip extensors is created by the deceleration of hip flexion during the swing phase and is assisted by ankle dorsiflexion. The tibialis anterior is contracted to lift the foot and, via the fibularis longus, draws down on the head of the fibula to further tension the biceps femoris, which is therefore pulled from both ends.
3. At heel strike, the deltoid of the hip uses the continuity between the latissimus dorsi and the opposite gluteus maximus with the ITB to help control and decelerate the pronation pattern created by the offset talus on the calcaneus.
4. The Deep Longitudinal Sling assists with the correction of the sacroiliac joints, using the continuity of the biceps femoris and the sacrotuberous ligament to apply a counter-nutation force to the SIJ on the side of the flexed leg, and using the opposite erector spinae and long dorsal sacroiliac ligament to create a nutation force acting on the SIJ on the side of the extended leg.
5. As the body progresses from weight acceptance to toe-off, the line of force at the greater trochanter switches from the gluteus maximus to the tensor fasciae latae, and the oblique line to the opposite shoulder girdle. This long anterior line of tension can be engaged to help with imminent hip flexion and to support supination of the foot prior to the propulsion.
6. The counterrotation in the upper thoracic spine that opposes the rotation driven from the pelvis is assisted by the upper shoulder girdle, thereby helping to stabilize the head. As the anterior obliques help in movement of the lower limb, the posterior rhomboids and splenii on that side will be shorter—and the reverse will be true on the other side of the body. This crossover in tension between the portions of the lines creates the counterrotation necessary for Gracovetsky's "Spinal Engine" and allows the skull to remain straight.
7. The essential events that allow us to take advantage of transverse plane efficiency mechanisms are: foot pronation and supination, nutation and counter-nutation of the sacroiliac joints, thoracic rotation, and contralateral arm swing.

6

OUR INNER SPRING

In walking, far from any vehicle or machine, from any mediation, I am replaying the earthly human condition, embodying once again man's inborn, essential destitution. That is why humility is not humiliating: it just makes vain pretensions fall away, and thus nudges us towards authenticity.

—Frédéric Gros, *A Philosophy of Walking*

■ INTRODUCTION

So far, we have focused on the superficial tissues in each plane and paid attention to myofascial continuities where the evidence supports them. Now we can dive into the more complex deeper tissues, which gives us an opportunity to draw each plane together simultaneously and to review our underpinning thesis that the body self-organizes tension levels to optimize efficiency. The body is wired to perceive the forces it is experiencing and to use that information to minimize eccentric and concentric contractions by using those forces to pre-tension the myofascial tissues. Whether those tissues are independent of one another or in series or in parallel, each tissue will have a role to play in the context of the body's shape as it progresses forward.

The shape the body makes is a result of skeletal alignment and the forces acting through it. Our movement pattern is not an accident—it has been honed over many millennia, and deviations from the ideal use will affect the tissues. Whether the extra work experienced by the muscles as a result of the deviations creates pain, tissue wear and tear, or any other form of pathology can be debated elsewhere; this book focuses on the efficiency of movement when all the necessary factors are in place. When those factors—almost any of the essential events—are awry, there are certain tissues that appear to be more affected than others (these tend to be the psoas, the quadratus lumborum, or the iliacus), but also our inner sense of "spring" is lost.

The inner blending of myofascia and visceral fascia that occurs throughout the body may be one reason why a walk in the country on a beautiful spring day feels so much easier than a winter's trudge to work. Our human condition allows us many different moods, and most are reflected in our body use. It may be the center of our being—the core—that makes the difference. For example, imagine your movement if you were to walk with a sense of depression or sadness. That internal deflation would rob something from the spring in your step. Some of that loss may be due to a shorter stride, as discussed earlier, but much will also result from the lower muscle tone and the loss of connection through the center of our bodies.

Although the continuity of many other myofascial lines has been challenged, few investigators have looked at the inner tissues of the so-called "Deep Front Line." With fascial tissues connecting the muscles of the jaw all the way to the soles of the feet via the neck, chest, abdomen, and pelvis, Myers' proposed Deep Front Line (DFL) is often referred to as the *core*. While this may be an overused and under-defined term, it does give a sense of the inner support that a toned and engaged Deep Front Line provides.[1] As we will see, the DFL may be used at both heel strike (hip flexion) and toe-off (hip extension); this occurs through the connections of the flexor and extensor adductors that stretch from the diaphragm through the pelvic floor to the feet.

The anatomy of Myers' DFL is more complex than the single plane tissues he proposed for the Superficial Front and Back Lines and the Lateral Line. Rather than presenting it as a line, Myers refers to it as a *volume*—something that fills the body's inner space of the torso and follows down the inside of the lower limb. The DFL includes tissues that manual therapists often find to be "tired," "overworked," "filled with trigger points," or hyper- or hypotonic. The adductors, iliacus and psoas, and quadratus lumborum all tend to fall into one of these categories.

In the previous chapters, I have tried to present an honest account of the anatomy of tissue continuity and where it may or may not overlap with everyday function. Wilke did not include the DFL as part of his meta-analysis, so there is less independent verification for the connections of tissues that Myers lists for this line. The lack of evidence means we have to work with an inner sense of the DFL rather than objective facts. In sensing it through the stretch positions outlined below, I hope you will experience the physical changes that the connections might bring; however, once again, the transfer of force may or may not be through the fascial tissues—that remains unproven. Whether or not it is through the fascial tissues is secondary to the reality of the movement pattern created to tension the anterior Deep Front Line, and that movement pattern corresponds to the extended toe-off position.

During toe-off we benefit from adequate pre-tensioning of the appropriate tissues and re-supination of the foot to create the rigid lever. Failure to achieve these ideal positions with the associated economies will initiate compensatory patterns that hamper the walking system. One feature of our species is the adaptive plasticity we demonstrate in movement strategies—we can walk with no toe extension, we can walk with limited side flexion, etc. But at what cost?

For example, to ideally stretch (i.e., pre-tension) the psoas (exercise 6.1), the leg would be positioned in extension, with abduction and medial rotation of the hip. The attentive reader will recognize that we have already covered these essential events in the sagittal, frontal, and transverse planes, and failure to achieve the position requires the recruitment of less-efficient movement strategies. The late Leon Chaitow often quoted "overuse, misuse, disuse and abuse" as the causes of soft-tissue dysfunction, and the question here is whether the inability to use momentum to properly pre-tension tissues prior to their use leads to the kind of symptoms described above. There are many reasons why one might not be able to pre-tension the deep tissues—in fact, all of them have already been listed—and it would be rare to find a client without some impairment in at least one of the essential events.

The overlap of essential events for the Deep Front Line and the previous planes affords us the opportunity to review many of the mechanisms and dynamics involved in gait. The repetition is useful, as we can now incorporate all the planes to embrace the complexity of the deeper tissues and come to each event with a slightly different view.

---

[1] By calling the DFL "engaged," I do not intend to invoke the conventional "core exercises" that deliberately contract the muscles, but refer instead to the mechanical engagement of the line that happens when appropriate movement allows the myofascia of the line to be stimulated.

■ THE INNER MECHANICS

In movement, the DFL (fig. 6.1) takes us in different directions using a number of "switches" or junctions. In the leg, the DFL begins with the three muscles of the deep posterior compartment and then crosses the medial aspect of the knee and divides into the anterior and posterior adductors. The myofascial divergence above the knee creates the switch that allows this line to be active in both hip flexion and extension, as the anterior adductors (pectineus, adductor brevis, and adductor longus) cross the front of the hip joint, and the posterior adductor (adductor magnus) crosses the back of the joint. From their respective attachments at the pelvis, the adductors will lead us into the pelvic, abdominal, and thoracic cavities, and finally come to the head via the hyoid complex and the throat.

The Deep Front Line certainly incorporates much of the intimate myofascia associated with inner support and vitality. Its fascia surrounds our viscera, the sensitive organs of the body, and is closely associated with our emotional states and even our sexuality. Many factors are involved in allowing this important line to play its diverse roles in movement. It requires balance with the more superficial myofascial tissues, which must be free enough to allow the tensional forces to travel to the deeper tissue (see fig. 6.2). Conversely, issues from within the DFL, such as internal health (whether emotional or structural) can be transferred to the outside, often forcing the outer lines to compensate for an impaired core.

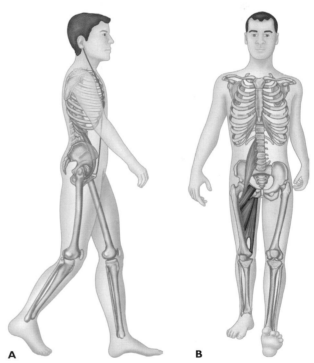

A   **B**

Figure 6.2.   *A, Any inability of the client to fully lengthen the superficial tissue, in this case the rectus femoris, prevents the mechanical tensioning of the psoas in the sagittal plane. B, This can lead to overuse issues, or it may lead to a compensation pattern in which the client uses external hip rotation to enlist the adductors for hip flexion.*

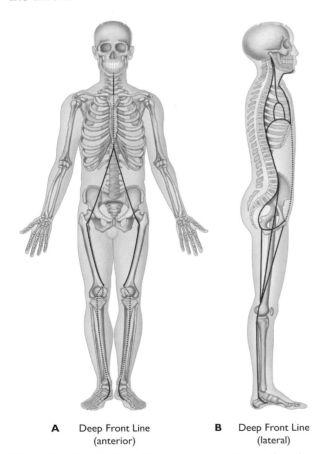

A   Deep Front Line   **B**   Deep Front Line
        (anterior)   (lateral)

Figure 6.1.   *The Deep Front Line takes us on a journey through the center of the body—anterior (A) and lateral (B) views. Often referred to as the "core," it is seen by many as being responsible for our inner support.*

The ability to see and recognize these patterns is important, as they can happen anywhere in the body, through any of the superficial tissues, preventing the mechanical load reaching deeper structures and inhibiting their ability to assist with the desired movement. Easy and graceful movement occurs when the superficial and deep tissues are able to work together, each doing their fair share of the work.

■ THE FOOT

The myofascia of the Deep Front Line is strongly associated with the support of the medial longitudinal arch and the midtarsal joints that make up the complex system within the foot. The tendons of the flexors hallucis and digitorum longus and tibialis posterior give us the final set of strings within a series of pulleys that work in concert to assist supination as part of the force-closure mechanism.

Each of the tendons of the deep posterior compartment wraps around the medial malleolus and dives under the sole of the foot. Of these, the flexor hallucis longus is especially important, as it threads its way below the sustentaculum tali, the promontory of the calcaneus supporting the talus. These three tendons also play an important role in preparing the foot for toe-off, by being tensioned in dorsiflexion (see fig. 6.3).

The fascia from the deep posterior compartment carries us over the medial aspect of the knee and onto the femur. From here, the tissue continues with the adductors. When considering pelvic tilts and shifts, we may need to address the adductors, as they can affect the position of the pelvis. But in the function of walking, the adductors convey the tensional changes from the pelvis to the medial longitudinal arch.

■ ANTERIOR INTERMUSCULAR SEPTUM

If we follow the anterior portion of the adductors from the medial epicondyle (the adductor tubercle), the fascial compartment will bring us toward the lesser trochanter via the adductors longus and brevis and the pectineus. These muscles attach to the pubic ramus, but their septal fascia will merge with that of the iliacus and psoas as their conjoined tendon crosses the front of the pelvis (Myers 2015). This anterior line therefore joins the inside of the foot to the diaphragm via three paths: the psoas, the quadratus lumborum and iliacus, and the pectineus and psoas minor (see fig. 6.4; Myers 2015).

■ POSTERIOR INTERMUSCULAR SEPTUM

If we return to the medial epicondyle, the posterior adductor septum will go to the ischiopubic ramus with the adductor magnus,

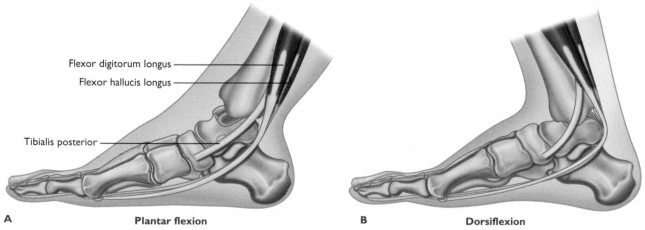

Flexor digitorum longus

Flexor hallucis longus

Tibialis posterior

A   **Plantar flexion**   **B**   **Dorsiflexion**

Figure 6.3.   *A, The three tendons of the deep posterior compartment all wrap around the back of the medial malleolus, which acts like a pulley—as the ankle dorsiflexes (B), the tendons will be tensioned, and they draw the bones of the foot together. It is almost like lacing your shoes: by pulling on the laces, you draw the sides of the shoe together, using the eyelets as the pulley. (See also fig. 6.9.)*

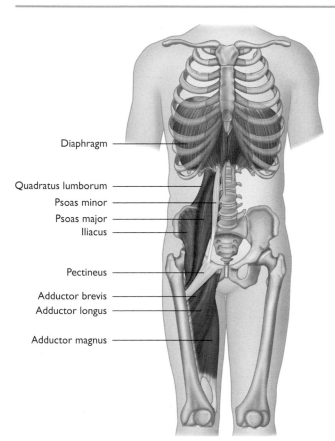

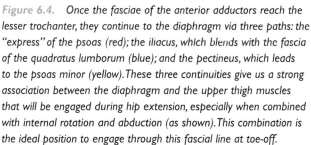

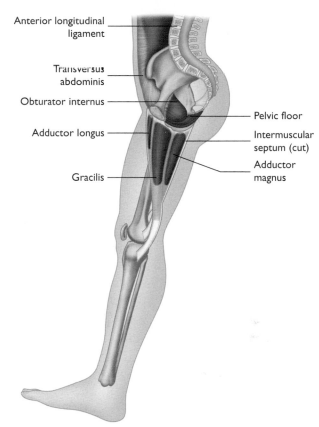

Figure 6.4. Once the fasciae of the anterior adductors reach the lesser trochanter, they continue to the diaphragm via three paths: the "express" of the psoas (red); the iliacus, which blends with the fascia of the quadratus lumborum (blue); and the pectineus, which leads to the psoas minor (yellow). These three continuities give us a strong association between the diaphragm and the upper thigh muscles that will be engaged during hip extension, especially when combined with internal rotation and abduction (as shown). This combination is the ideal position to engage through this fascial line at toe-off.

Figure 6.5. The posterior intermuscular septum will bring us along the adductor magnus to the ischiopubic ramus, blending into the obturator internus and from there to the pelvic floor. The continuity from the pelvic floor can also go in two directions—anteriorly, with the transversus abdominis, or along the front of the spine, with the anterior longitudinal ligament. Both of these tracks will bring us to the cranium.

which blends into the fascia of the obturator internus and, thereby, to the pelvic floor. From the pelvic floor, the myofascial continuity continues to the head via the anterior longitudinal ligament or the deep aspect of the transversus abdominis, which blends with the abdominal and thoracic intracavity linings, leading us into the throat to reach the cranium (see fig. 6.5; Myers 2015). As we will see later in this chapter, the tensioning of the posterior line in the thigh is important for "core" support at heel strike.

Much of the inner support for the head may come from the tissues of the Deep Front Line. If we continue the line from the back of the transversus abdominis, it brings us to the tissue

on the back of the sternum and eventually upward to the infrahyoids and suprahyoids. Many of the deep anterior supporting muscles of the neck, such as the longus capitis and colli (see fig. 6.6), are a continuation of tissues ascending from the diaphragm, which we reached via the psoas and quadratus lumborum. Therefore, if the head is correctly placed on the top of the cervical spine and supported by the muscles ascending from the thoracic cage, in balance with the erectors, the superficial tissues of the shoulder muscles should be free to perform their duties for the shoulders—if we are standing still. However, as we will see in chapter 7, once we begin to move, the head becomes a very heavy and potentially unstable unit on top of a slender pole of support. In function, therefore, the head

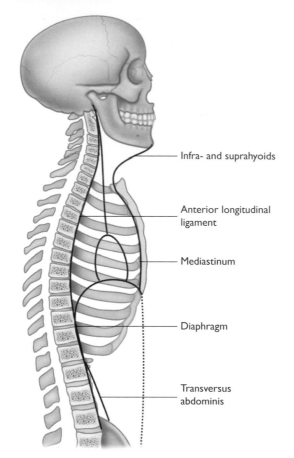

- Infra- and suprahyoids
- Anterior longitudinal ligament
- Mediastinum
- Diaphragm
- Transversus abdominis

Figure 6.6. The Deep Front Line incorporates much (if not all) of our internal visceral fascia. For our purposes, however, we follow the three main myofascial lines described by Myers (2015) to reach the front of the cranium—the hyoids leading to the muscles of the jaw, the muscles supporting the front of the neck, and the anterior longitudinal ligament leading to the foramen magnum.

requires the extra lines of tension coming from superficial tissues, especially those connecting it to the shoulders.

■ DEEP FRONT LINE— PRONATION TO SUPINATION

In the preparation for toe-off, the medial longitudinal arch should correct from pronation, allowing the midtarsal joints to reengage and create a more stable foot to launch from. A number of mechanisms will be involved in this procedure, one through the bones and two via the soft tissue. It is the action of the swing leg coming through into flexion that stimulates each of these mechanisms. As we saw in the sagittal plane (chapter 3),

the swing leg causes a rotation of the pelvis to the opposite side, which laterally rotates the supporting femur (the stance leg). This rotation will encourage the tibia and the fibula to rotate in the same direction. Held as it is in the mortise between the malleoli, the talus will also turn, lifting the calcaneus with it (as described in chapter 2).

This mechanism of the bones is supported by the obliquely oriented soft tissues (chapter 5). Once the leg comes into extension, the line of tissue from the tensor fasciae latae to the tibialis anterior will be pulled, lifting the base of the first metatarsal, the top of the foot's dome. When the hip joint is in extension, internal rotation, and abduction—the ideal position for tensioning of the psoas, iliacus, and anterior adductors—it tensions the Deep Front Line prior to toe-off and assists force closure. At the same time, the ankle is dorsiflexed and the knee extended, a position that potentially engages the anterior DFL all the way from the neck to the inside of the foot, but especially from the diaphragm through the psoas (see exercise 6.1 and figs. 6.7 & 6.8).

Exercise 6.1. Step forward with one leg, keeping the heel of the back foot on the floor. Internally rotate your back leg slightly and then slowly bring your pelvis into a posterior tilt or experiment with shifting it horizontally forward and back slightly. Can you feel the medial arch lift slightly as you tilt back and/or as you bring the pelvis forward? Can you feel the connection from the front of the pelvis across the inside of the back of the knee to the medial arch? You may feel a stretch along the anterior septum of the thigh, the inside of the knee, or even along the medial aspect of the tibia, but wherever the sensation is, it will be somewhere along this strong fascial line of the anterior DFL (unless the tightness of the calf prevents you from achieving the position!).

The Z-shaped stretch that is created in the DFL prior to toe-off complements the

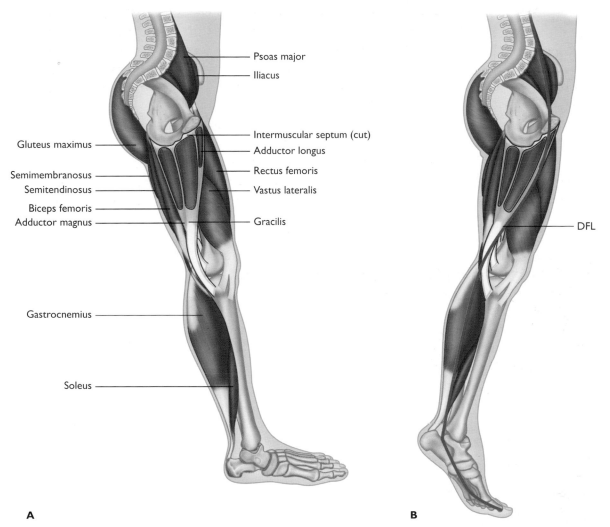

Psoas major
Iliacus
Intermuscular septum (cut)
Adductor longus
Rectus femoris
Vastus lateralis
Gracilis
Gluteus maximus
Semimembranosus
Semitendinosus
Biceps femoris
Adductor magnus
Gastrocnemius
Soleus
DFL

A   B

Figure 6.7.   A, Immediately after heel strike, the anterior portion of the Deep Front Line adductors will be disengaged—because of hip and knee flexion—allowing the foot to pronate in response to the ground reaction force. B, As we come into hip extension, knee extension, ankle dorsiflexion, and toe extension, the DFL line comes into a Z-shaped stretch as the tissue wraps around the pulleys of the front of the pubic ramus and the back of the medial malleolus.

actions of the oblique tissues. The tissue of the tibialis anterior will be drawn up by the extension occurring at the hip and by the lateral rotation of the tibia, lifting the base of the first metatarsal. The fibularis longus and brevis will be tensioned by the dorsiflexion of the ankle, as they wrap around the lateral malleolus. The fibularis longus will meet and further support the tibialis anterior, combining their efforts to stabilize the mobile first ray (see fig. 6.9).

As the ankle dorsiflexes, the fibularis brevis will draw the fifth metatarsal into the cuboid to provide lateral stability, but it—and its longer compatriot—must be in balance with

the medial tissues of the DFL and allow the ankle to dorsiflex evenly. A common pattern is for the lateral band of the plantar fascia or the fibularis tendons to be short, which causes them to hold the foot in a lateral rotation. This prevents the corrective supination of the foot that should occur in order to engage the midtarsal joints.

As we saw above, the prime supporters of the midtarsal complex are the tendons of the deep posterior compartment: tibialis posterior, flexor hallucis longus, and flexor digitorum longus. The flexor hallucis longus clearly helps lift the proximal part of the arch by supporting the sustentaculum tali. It then provides a tension wire along the entire medial aspect of the foot to the big toe, which also dorsiflexes as the foot progresses onto the toe rocker, further lengthening the DFL line. The flexor hallucis longus is also crossed by the flexor digitorum longus, giving a suspension to the arch, especially during the toe rocker phase (see fig. 6.9).

The tibialis posterior is the last part of the supporting and balancing system of the foot from the lower leg. Its tendon attaches to all

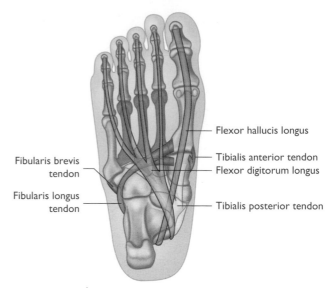

Figure 6.9.   *The long tendons attaching to the plantar surface create a corrective system for the arches of the foot. The tibialis anterior and fibularis longus (red) form a sling. While they usually work in opposition to one another, they do cooperate to draw the base of the first metatarsal into the medial arch. The fibularis brevis does the same for the fifth metatarsal and the lateral arch.*

the middle metatarsals—second, third, and fourth—as well as to the bones comprising the bulk of the midtarsal joint complex: the navicular, all three cuneiforms, and the cuboid. So, while the other tendons give distal (the two long toe flexors), medial (the tibialis anterior and fibularis longus), and lateral (the fibularis brevis) support, it is really the tibialis posterior that draws the central and more stable bones together (see fig. 6.9).

The tibialis posterior is challenged, however, by the positioning of its flat tendon under the malleolus, as this is an area of high stress at heel strike, which requires the absorption of the forceful rear foot eversion. This section of the tendon is hypovascular, and dysfunction can greatly affect the mechanics of the rest of the foot (and therefore the rest of the body!) and can be slow and stubborn to correct.

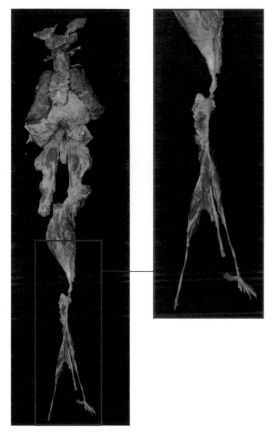

Figure 6.8.   *A fresh tissue dissection supports the presence of the strong myofascial connection from the front of the pelvis to the inside of the foot.[1] Note the strong tendinous element between the medial epicondyle, along the medial aspect of the knee joint to the popliteus and into the deep posterior compartment (shown in inset). Many people feel this section "pull" when doing exercise 6.1, and the orientation of the fibers shows that it is more involved in this vertical transfer of force from walking than with the oblique pull from the popliteus, with which it is continuous. (Image courtesy of Anatomy Trains.)*

Referring to fig. 6.9, the two long toe flexors, hallucis and digitorum longus (*blue*), cross under the medial arch. As they are tensioned by the combined dorsiflexion of the ankle and toe rockers, they support and

---

[1]It should be noted that the ability to dissect myofascial continuities is only supportive evidence for their existence; it does not prove their use or their ability to transfer force.

"approximate" (pull together) the distal ends, or at least they prevent them from spreading further away.

The tibialis posterior (*yellow*) attaches to almost everything else, including the navicular, all three cuneiforms, and the cuboid, and it gives support to the three metatarsals not supported by the tibialis anterior or fibularis brevis. This strong corrector of pronation therefore crosses the midtarsal and tarsometatarsal joints of the second to fourth rays (*green*). These tarsometatarsal joints only allow dorsiflexion/plantar flexion; the first and fifth (*uncolored*) have more variation in their movements and are stabilized differently to allow this flexibility.

■ TOE-OFF

Once the foot is brought back to the supinated position through the combination of inversion, lateral rotation, and dorsiflexion, the bones create a stable base to push from. In relaxed

walking, however, we very rarely "push" during toe-off; instead, we use most of the so-called "plantar flexors" in isometric contraction, as we saw with the gastrocnemius and soleus. So, while these tissues may be lengthening proximally in dorsiflexion, they are shortening distally to bring together the bones of the feet (the "econcentric" action described in chapter 5). This form of contraction is necessary, as the proximal portions of all of these myofascial elements will be moving away from the distal insertions as the leg tilts forward to create the dorsiflexion (see fig. 6.10).

Mechanoreceptors—the Internal Monitors

We actively "push off" when we need to walk faster or ascend a slope. At those times, the tension is constantly monitored and adjusted through the mechanoreceptors in the calf. In an ingenious experiment, Sawicki applied a mechanical boot with pneumatic "muscles" that assisted plantar flexion (Sawicki, Lewis,

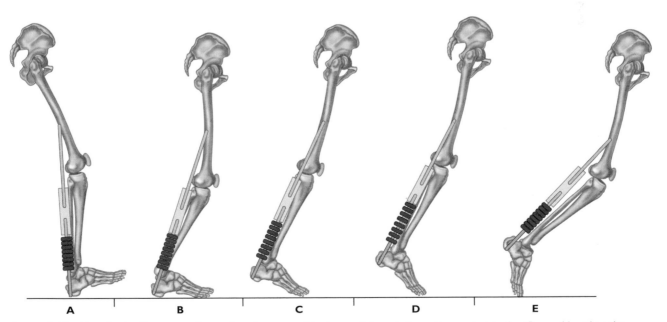

Figure 6.10. *From heel strike, as we roll over the calcaneus and begin to roll through the ankle, we start to dorsiflex and lengthen the plantar flexors (A and B). This decelerates the lower leg, allowing the femur to move faster, with the swing of the other leg, and bring the knee into extension, as we roll onto the ball of the foot (C). Coming into toe dorsiflexion with the toe rocker (D) creates the final portion of the wind-up in the elastic tissue, which is released like a catapult mechanism in toe-off (E).*

and Ferris 2009). It gave "free" energy to the subject's toe-off phase, and the research team found that users quickly altered the amount of muscle force they used in order to adapt and compensate for the extra force coming from the boot. This allowed the subject to keep their walking kinematics relatively normal. "The user's nervous system reduced the triceps surae muscle activity in response to the mechanical assistance." Essentially, the demands of the job changed, and the mechanoreceptors adjusted the muscle effort accordingly.

What Sawicki, Lewis, and Ferris are saying is that our internal mechanoreceptors are able to constantly adjust in accordance with the mechanical forces involved in walking, keeping the muscle activity at a minimum to ensure maximum efficiency. Sawicki continued to explore the benefits of muscle architecture that allow this elastic mechanism and found that they tend to be pennate muscles with long tendons (see fig. 6.11). Pennate muscles—in which the muscle fibers are attached to the tendons at an angle—allow a greater number of fibers to be included in the muscle unit. This in turn allows a muscle to create more power, or, in the case of the triceps surae, allows it to withstand more lengthening, so that the kinetic force goes into and loads the elastic tissues of the tendons (and the surrounding fascial elements).

Sawicki, Lewis, and Ferris used surface EMG and focused their readings on the soleus muscle, but looking at the architecture of the plantar flexors of the deep posterior compartment we can clearly see that they all follow the same pattern of pennation with long tendons (see fig. 6.11). This interrelationship between muscle fiber arrangement and percentage of collagenous tissues, and the architectural relationship of the fibers in context with the functional roles of each muscle brings us back to the arrangements we saw in fig. 1.26. Fig. 1.26 illustrates the length force–length relationship relative to the stage at which the collagenous (passive) tissue begins

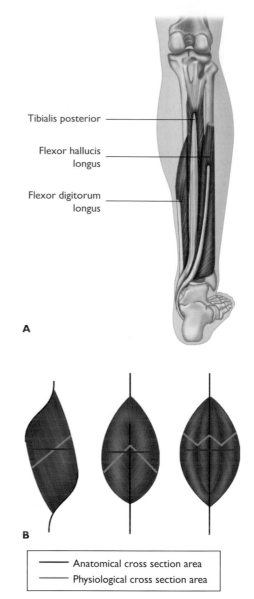

Tibialis posterior

Flexor hallucis longus

Flexor digitorum longus

A

B

—— Anatomical cross section area
—— Physiological cross section area

Figure 6.11. In the anatomy of the deep posterior calf muscles (A), we can see the angulation of the muscle fibers and their long, elastic tendons diving under the foot to join the phalanges and the tarsals. This arrangement means the muscles have a shorter range of motion than a fusiform muscle (a muscle with fibers that are parallel and run the full length of the unit). In cross section (B), we can see how we have to take a series of sections of a pennate muscle to count the actual number of fibers contained in a single unit, compared to the fusiform muscle, for which only one section is needed. The result of this is that the fusiform muscles have a longer range but produce less power than the shorter-range pennate muscles. In the case of our leg muscles, that power is used to encourage the kinetic energy to load the elastic fascial tissues. By holding isometric contractions, the muscle saves metabolic energy and stores kinetic energy for use in the catapult system.

to strain and assist with control of movement. Combining our understanding of the fiber direction, the deceleration of momentum, and the gait phase at which each muscle is recruited gives an enhanced appreciation of form and function relationships.

The dorsiflexors perform a considerable amount of work in the deceleration of forward momentum and the lift of the stable foot as the body progresses from heel strike to toe-off. Greater joint ranges are experienced at the foot and ankle than at the hip and knee, both of which are supported by passive structures at their extremes of extension (the iliofemoral ligament and the patella, respectively). This contrasts with the foot and ankle, which do not reach their full passive range during normal gait and therefore require active myofascial support. Long, strong tendons which strain in short ranges, controlled by pennate muscles and placed in areas of high momentum, therefore make functional sense for the calf.

THE COMBINED POWER OF HIP EXTENSION AND ANKLE DORSIFLEXION

As mentioned earlier, a Z-shaped stretch that pre-tensions the Deep Front Line is created by combining foot dorsiflexion and hip extension, and in exercise 6.1 one can feel the connection from the front of the pelvis to the medial arch of the foot. One can also feel the connection from the pelvis up through the upper body— see exercise 6.2 below. The Deep Front Line is pre-tensioned through the position created by momentum in each plane, which is why we have left it until now to explore.

Exercise 6.2. **Start by assuming the same position as in exercise 6.1—one leg back and internally rotated—and bring yourself to the "point of bind," where the medial arch of the back foot begins to lift.**

Now bring your body into a gentle thoracic extension, so that your rib cage is up, but then exhale deeply to help relax the scalenes and the deep anterior neck tissue. Do you sense a

change through the center of your body? Does it affect your back foot and its arch?

With this exercise, you can also explore the effects of the different movements. More of one will restrict the other—for example, more thoracic extension may limit your ability to internally rotate your hip. Similarly, and perhaps more concerning, if there is not enough "loading" in one plane, then another movement must be increased to compensate. A decrease in adduction or abduction may increase the need for extension, or for more work to be produced by the muscles involved.

The implication of this phenomenon is that too much movement in one plane may also limit the loading of tissues in another plane, while too little loading in one plane will increase the movement required in another— that is, insufficient loading, causing a lack of elastic recoil, will require more work from the muscles to aid the recovery. This is a central part of this book's thesis: the movements that occur to lengthen the fascial tissue must be balanced. The most efficient combination of movements is a "Goldilocks" event, with just the right amount of movement and load. This is true for all of the other areas we have looked at so far, and we will discuss this in more detail in chapter 8.

UNRAVELING THE PSOAS

The psoas is perhaps the muscle with the most conflicting descriptions—it is variously described as a strong hip flexor or not a hip flexor at all, an internal or external rotator, and an adductor or abductor of the hip. The truth is that it will do all of these things, depending on your starting position. When describing function, we must not limit ourselves to discussions based on anatomical position and the concentric/ eccentric model of movement—the body is much more interesting than that. Unfortunately, it can be much more confusing too.

Gibbons (in Vleeming et al. 2007) summarizes much of the work that has been done on the function of the psoas in an attempt to gain some clarity. Most investigations have shown the psoas to have little effect in movement of the lumbar spine, except perhaps in the production of lordosis; however, it has quite consistently been found to create axial compression of the lumbar spine, meaning that when tensioned, the psoas helps stabilize the lower spinal segments. Gibbons also describes the fascial anatomy of the psoas as being continuous into the tissues of the transversus abdominis, internal oblique, and pelvic floor, again emphasizing its potential role within this "core stability" complex.

Interestingly, Gibbons describes the psoas as being a unipennate muscle (i.e., it has one group of pennate, angled fibers) with shorter than expected muscle fibers, which makes him question "its efficiency as a hip flexor," as the fibers show no significant change of length. He posits that the iliacus is a more active flexor of the hip joint. However, there may be a different interpretation of this information. As we saw above with the three tendons of the deep posterior compartment and the work of Sawicki, efficiency is increased by having a pennate structure. As the hip goes into extension, the muscle tissue of the psoas may be contracting to send the load into the elastic tissues, which will then recoil into flexion. At the same time, the mechanism will encourage a "force closure" of the lumbars. Compressing the lumbars as the hip goes into extension appears functionally sound, since it will increase the stability of the lower back as the body's center of gravity moves away from its base of support.

It therefore seems that the Z-stretch created in hip extension/ankle dorsiflexion assists a force-closure form of stability at both ends of this line (see fig. 6.12). Combining the use of momentum and pennate muscles, the Z-position helps draw together the loose bones of the foot and stabilize the vulnerable lumbar spine in preparation for toe-off.

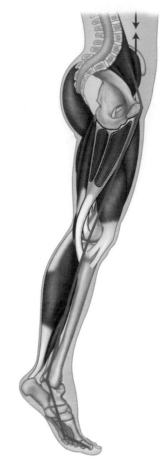

Figure 6.12. *In this deliberately exaggerated view, you can see how the Z-stretch begins to draw together the less-stable bones of both the foot and the lumbar spine to create a force-closure effect and to produce a more stable platform for toe-off.*

■ DEEP FRONT LINE AT HEEL STRIKE AND A HEALTHY PELVIC FLOOR

The calcaneus prepares itself for heel strike by slightly inverting in the moments before the foot contacts the ground. Some of this is achieved by tensioning the tibialis anterior, but that muscle's attachments on the base of the first metatarsal are quite far from the calcaneus, indicating there is perhaps another mechanism at work in the calcaneus's movement. This may involve a reciprocal line of tension in the deep posterior compartment.

The fascia crossing the medial aspect of the knee may be able to communicate tension from both the flexor and extensor adductors to the foot, allowing them to create some foot supination (see fig. 6.13). However, this is speculative and currently unsupported within the literature. At heel strike, if the connection does exist, it is very quickly lost, as the foot rapidly plantar flexes, the knee flexes, and the hip adducts. All of those movements will break the tension in the fascial continuity, despite the strong contraction of the adductor magnus.

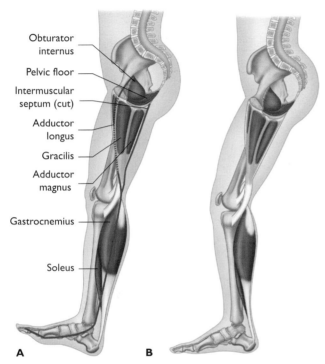

Figure 6.13. *A, Prior to heel strike, the posterior section of the DFL is tensioned via the combination of hip flexion, knee extension, and foot dorsiflexion, which allows the tissue of the adductor magnus to communicate to the myofascia supporting the medial arch. B, Heel strike causes rapid plantar flexion, knee flexion, and hip adduction (not shown here), all of which reduce the fascial communication across the joints.*

The adductor magnus assists the hamstrings, the gluteus maximus, and the other hip extensors at heel strike. Its fascial continuity, however, is with the obturator internus on the other side of the ischiopubic ramus, which gives us another strategy to decelerate the internal rotation of the femur. This could prove an interesting subject of future research: to look at the relationship between these two muscles, which work together to stabilize the pelvis in flexion but which oppose each another in rotation.

Following heel strike, the mechanical stimulus from the adductor magnus and obturator internus may carry tension to the pelvic floor and thus to the psoas, through its continuity with the transversus abdominis. Therefore, the adductor magnus may also be able to "switch on" the "core" system, especially in the pelvic floor. This is seen in the way the pelvic floor is initially tonified by an infant's many teetering experiments while learning to walk (see fig. 6.14).

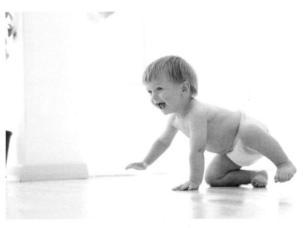

Figure 6.14. *In the wobbling, unsteady process of the first attempts at walking, a toddler uses the adductors, which stimulates contractions and tone in the pelvic floor. This not only helps the child learn to stand and walk but also helps him or her to establish urinary and fecal continence.*

By stimulating a contraction within the walls of muscle that surround the abdominopelvic cavity (the pelvic floor, the transversus abdominis, and the diaphragm), the body may take advantage of another hydraulic amplifier mechanism (see fig. 6.15). Although this may be difficult to visualize in its three dimensions, we have to consider the implications of the cavity's volume and the various pressures and tensions involved during movement. The arrangement also demonstrates the significance of in-series and in-parallel tensioning mechanisms. Through tensioning the transversus abdominis, the body pre-tensions the epimysia—the sheath of tissue surrounding individual muscles—of the muscles that stabilize the lower back: the psoas, quadratus lumborum, erector spinae,

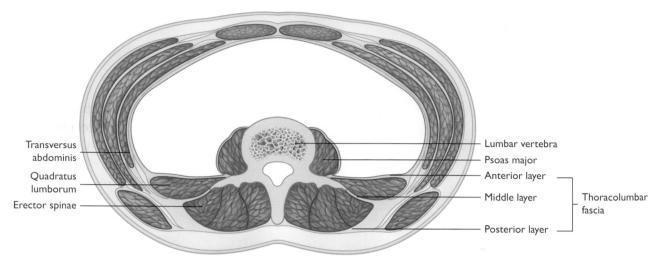

Labels: Transversus abdominis, Quadratus lumborum, Erector spinae, Lumbar vertebra, Psoas major, Anterior layer, Middle layer, Posterior layer, Thoracolumbar fascia

Figure 6.15.   *The contraction of the adductor magnus at heel strike may stimulate the pelvic floor and transversus abdominis, tensioning the fascial layers surrounding the erector spinae, helping to stabilize the lower back and assisting the erectors.*

and multifidi. These different layers of muscle may be receiving mechanical tension via different layers of the thoracolumbar fascia (TLF): the psoas via the transversus abdominis and the anterior and middle layers of the TLF; the quadratus lumborum and multifidi via the middle layers; and the erector spinae also from the middle layer. All of the muscles are given compressional support from the superficial layer through its connections to the latissimus dorsi and gluteus maximus.

FRONT AND BACK BALANCING

The posterior layer of the important thoracolumbar fascia is also the connection between the latissimus dorsi on one side of the body and the gluteus maximus on the opposite side, as discussed in chapter 5.

The latissimus dorsi and gluteus maximus form the posterior section of the "swingwalker" mechanism proposed by Zorn and Hodeck. In this model, Zorn and Hodeck (in Dalton 2011) suggest that an "inverted pendulum" model of gait requires the efficiency of elastic recoil on the front and back of the body (see fig. 6.16). As discussed earlier, the front of

the body contributes significantly through the sagittally and obliquely oriented abdominals. Both of these planes, however, are quite superficial, taking us from the pelvis to the thoracic cage. By tensioning the psoas prior to toe-off, we can follow a more profound path, bringing us to the inside of the ilium and the anterior lumbar spine, and connecting to the diaphragm via this internal route.

> We created a sagittal plane model in a computer program and endowed it with the precise anthropometric data…. We solved the movement equations with the help of some mathematical tools of applied mechanics and determined the spring parameters (length and stiffness) that make the design work properly.
>
> —Zorn and Hodeck, in Dalton (2011)

The three-dimensional network of connective tissue, so richly endowed with mechanoreceptors, is the body's computer network. It is constantly receiving stimulation through movement, and—presumably through pattern recognition—it can adjust the muscle tone to make the correct response.

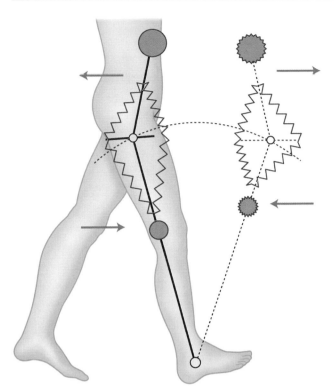

Figure 6.16. Rolfers and physicists Adjo Zorn and Kai Hodeck developed a computer-based model of walking. Expanding on previous works that looked at walking as a pendulum-type action, they realized the necessity of adding a second—and inverted—pendulum connected with two springs. If they correctly set the tension in the springs, the model was able to turn kinetic energy into elastic energy and thus produce a passive system of movement that required no engine (muscle) or other form of energy. (Adapted from Zorn and Hodeck, in Dalton 2011.)

Through repetition (how many times does a toddler fall down before he or she learns how to stand up, then cruise, then walk, then run?), it seems we learn the most efficient methods of moving.

Zorn and Hodeck suggest that the psoas in particular is the elastic element in efficient movement that works in opposition to the posterior sling. The psoas is often greatly honored by bodyworkers and movement therapists for its central role within the body and for the fact that it acts as a conduit for the lumbar plexus. However, I feel that the overworked psoas is one of a collection of tissues that has to compensate a little harder when it is not effectively pre-tensioned, and this is the reason that it may become dysfunctional in some way.

As we saw above, the psoas crosses the hip and all of the lumbar joints and has a number of roles to play in the balance between mobility and stability. As a hip flexor, adductor, and internal rotator, it should be optimally loaded in the final position prior to toe-off. In the toe-off position, the hip should be extended, abducted, and medially rotated; failing to achieve tensioning in any of those planes (sagittal extension, frontal plane abduction, or transverse plane rotation) may necessitate concentric contractions of the psoas to compensate and may lead to overwork. The ability to reach the correct position in each plane is, of course, not isolated to the functioning of the hip, but is dependent on many other joints through the lower limb on the same side as well as the opposite lower limb and the lumbar and thoracic spines. This explains the emphasis on the "essential events" listed throughout this text, as failing to achieve them will require the deeper tissues to compensate.

▪ ELASTIC EFFICIENCY MONITORING

Zorn and Hodeck's work gives us a valid (though computer-generated) model for how the body might be able to take advantage of reciprocal arrangements to encourage the efficiency of elastic recoil. Obviously, it is much more complex than the pelvis being able to bounce back and forth on a computer screen. However, the quote above can give us insight into the mechanical monitoring process that we saw earlier in Sawicki's mechanical plantar flexing boot, in which the plantar flexors adjusted the strength of their firing in concert with the work that was being produced by the boot. When plantar flexion was assisted, the muscles somehow "knew" to do less work.

We see this kind of internal and automatic adjustment occurring in other studies, such as ones that examined the force of heel strike with various amounts of cushioning. Essentially, the degree of protection offered to the foot changes the amount of force with which the foot hits the ground. This is what you can feel if you start using shoes with less cushioning after a few days of wearing more protective shoes: the first few steps are harder than normal. But the body quickly adapts, equalizing the forces with no conscious effort on your part.

Research by Snel (cited in Gracovetsky, in Dalton 2011) shows that the forces at impact remain relatively stable regardless of the footwear used (see fig. 6.17). While the study looked at running, it may also inform us about the change in heel strike impact following a sudden switch of footwear. Quite often when transitioning from cushioned to thinner soles, one can feel the shock of the heel strike for the first step or two, as the "computations" recalibrate the absorbing system.

A number of reasons have been put forward for this. I believe the transition period allows us to optimize the amount of kinetic loading we receive into the body. If we land with too much force, the body cannot effectively absorb the shock; if we land too softly, the deceleration force required to absorb the shock is not strong enough to load the elastic tissue, forcing the body to use more energy to continue its

movement—it is more energy inefficient to creep than to walk. And so, when working properly, the mechanoreceptors are looking for that "Goldilocks" level at which the kinetic energy is "just right" to load the elastic tissue and benefit from the elastic recoil to reduce active work.

Postural Considerations

Maintaining an upright stance influences tissue pre-tension in a positive way. The connections from the jaw and throat into the thoracic cavity and onto the diaphragm seem able to create a proximal tensioning of the hip flexors. The sprinter Michael Johnson ran with his back extended and his chin tucked in, apparently taking advantage—to great effect—of the extra recoil available from the anterior tissues (see fig. 6.18).

An anterior head position, a collapsed rib cage, and any rotations and tilts in the spine may all negatively influence the flow of tensions in the front of the body, which will contribute to imbalances. The task is to learn to identify these postural problems and to make the appropriate changes through directed interventions—exercise, stretching, and soft-tissue manipulation, as necessary.

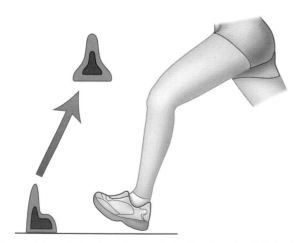

Figure 6.17. When investigating the heel strike pulse (P1), Snel showed that using a variation of footwear with different paddings (as well as being barefoot) made very little difference to the heel strike pulse. It was proposed that the body adjusts its movement to maintain a relatively consistent loading through the tissue.

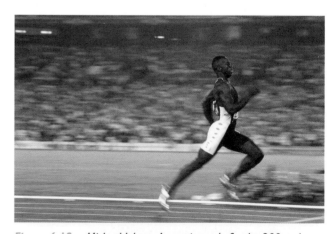

Figure 6.18. Michael Johnson's running style for the 200 and 400 meters was revolutionary at the time. His upright stance, combined with shorter strides, was perhaps maximizing the elastic recoil through the Deep Front Line to speed hip flexion. (Photograph courtesy of Getty Images.)

■ ESSENTIAL EVENTS

As the previous chapters have already covered each of the three planes of motion—sagittal, frontal, and transverse—most of the events are now accounted for. There is only one essential event, outlined below, specific to the Deep Front Line, but the important point for the deeper tissues is that all of the superficial tissues are able to load simultaneously.

Our aim should be to ensure an even load through each tissue so that no one tissue has to produce more work or absorb more stress than any other. Superficial tissues must be long enough to let the momentum of movement load the deeper tissues; they also must be strong enough to absorb their fair share of the forces involved. Dysfunction will result from imbalances in the "stiffness absorbing system" of the myofascia, caused by overuse or underuse. To correct dysfunction, one must find ways of using strengthening and stretching exercises that target the appropriate tissue, while also recognizing the role of the mechanoreceptors; not all dysfunction is caused by tissue limitations—it can be caused by motor patterning.

Gently encouraging clients into the essential events can tell you whether movement restrictions are proprioceptive or actual tissue limitations. We often learn bad habits, failing to use the full length of our myofascia through movement patterns caused by previous injuries or simply by mimicking (consciously and unconsciously) the movement of someone close to us. These bad habits can train our mechanoreceptors to use patterns that are not ideal for fascial efficiency, requiring more work and/or creating imbalance at the transition points of heel strike and toe-off.

Z-Stretch and Hip Position

As you felt in the two exercises in this chapter (6.1 and 6.2), the engagement of the deep hip flexors plays an important role at the point of toe-off. For a fully effective engagement of the psoas tendon, the psoas needs to be properly elongated, a position achieved by the extended hip being abducted and internally rotated relative to the pelvis. Not only is the tendon's distal attachment being lengthened, but the proximal attachment on the diaphragm will also be side flexing to the opposite side (see fig. 6.19).

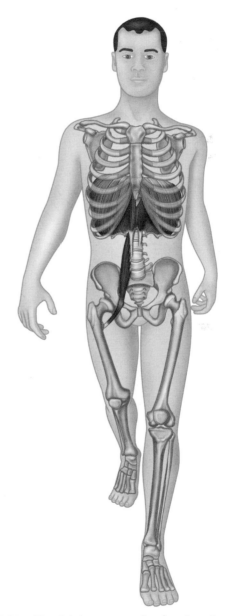

Figure 6.19. *This slightly exaggerated outline shows how the hip and lumbar movements conspire to allow full elastic loading of the psoas tendon. As discussed in the psoas section earlier, not only will this assist with toe-off, but it may also contribute to lumbar stability, important in those moments of greatest challenge, at the extreme ends of normal range. The psoas manages to perform two tasks in one movement—the countermovement of the lower limb and the stabilization of the lower back.*

In the ideal extended position for toe-off, we could list the essential events as:

- Toe extension
- Knee extension
- Hip extension, abduction, and internal rotation (same side)
- Hip flexion, adduction, and external rotation (opposite side)
- Heel strike and knee extension (opposite side)
- Sacroiliac nutation (same side) and counter-nutation (opposite side)
- Relative rotation between the thorax and the pelvis
- Spinal extension
- Contralateral arm swing
- Thoracic rotation

■ SUMMARY

1. Force transfer through the Deep Front Line has not been proven but implications of its continuity can be felt in the Z-position stretch, which mimics the body's position at toe-off.
2. The ideal pre-tension position for the DFL matches that for the other planes.
3. Momentum is controlled by the pennate muscles of the deep posterior compartment and psoas. The use of pennation assists the control of high strain forces entering the fascial tissues.
4. Tension levels are unconsciously optimized in response to the forces acting through the body.
5. Failure to achieve the ideal pre-tensioning leads to the potential for overuse, misuse, and disuse of various tissues.

7

CONTRALATERAL MOVEMENT

If we select any object from the
whole extent of animated nature,
and contemplate it fully and in all its
bearings, we shall certainly come to this
conclusion: that there is design in the
mechanical construction, benevolence
in the endowments of the living
properties, and that good on the whole
is the result.

—Charles Bell, 1837, *The Hand: Its
Mechanisms and Vital Endowments as
Evincing Design*

■ INTRODUCTION

The role of the upper limbs during gait is
debated—are they passive dampers for the
rotational forces driven up from the turn of
the pelvis or are they active contributors to
walking? Research findings have been equivocal
and so we are left to explore many of the aspects
for ourselves. Like the way college essays
are compared and contrasted by many, our
conclusion is that the upper limbs are capable of
both and that both are useful contributions.

The upper girdles respond to the movement
coming up from the lower body and provide

a form of counterweight to it that may assist
in damping the rotational force passing
above and in containing it below. The idea
of damping may therefore distract from how
the girdles also contribute as a form of trigger
mechanism. The foot's anchor to the ground
allows tension to build up in the tissues above
the foot as the body moves over it. Without
that anchor, the tensional force would be
lost or never build up in the first place. The
counterrotational ability of the shoulder
complex may perform a similar anchoring
role for transverse plane movement. The
counterweight of the shoulders adds stability
to the body by containing rather than damping
the forces—they provide the counterforce
similar to that when we wring a dishrag.
Turning the cloth with just one hand will not
build tension in the fibers—it requires hands at
either end and at least one turning to create the
wringing effect.

Chapter 5 explored transverse plane movement
through the lower limbs and trunk, and,
while we have mentioned the oblique slings
previously, we will explore them now in more
detail. The slings/lines of Vleeming and Myers
connect the shoulder complexes to the opposite
lower limbs on the front and back, giving us
contralateral tissues to exploit our natural
contralateral movement.

Designed by Time

Whether we see the body as evolved or designed (as Charles Bell did), I think we would all agree on the wonderful job done on the upper limb. The dexterity of the hand and the range of motion of the shoulder are both excellent schemes, allowing so many of our human abilities.

A contemporary of Bell's, Richard Lovejoy, is credited with being the first to notice that the schema for upper and lower limbs are virtually identical. And, as any visitor to the Natural History Museum in London (which Lovejoy founded), will see, this is not exclusive to humans: just about every other animal that has limbs follows a similar pattern—scapula/pelvis, humerus/femur, ulna and radius/tibia and

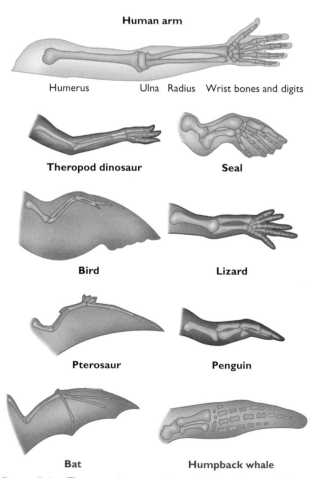

Figure 7.1. *The general pattern of upper-limb architecture follows a similar pattern of one bone, then two, followed by a series of smaller bones in various arrangements.*

fibula. There is much more variation in the carpals, tarsals, and phalanges, depending on the digitation strategy (hoofed, webbed, fingered, and so forth), but the overall building blocks are the same (see fig. 7.1).

Paleontologist Neil Shubin recently published his work on the discovery of Tiktaalik, a fossil found in 2004 on Ellesmere Island, Canada, and dated to 375 million years ago (see fig. 7.2). Tiktaalik is significant, as it is a transition fossil, the remains of an amphibian that had the beginnings of jointed arms and a cervical spine. On the basis of his study of other specimens, Shubin had predicted that these features should be found in fossils from approximately 375 MYA. After hunting down geological areas that would have encountered the correct weather patterns at that period, he found Tiktaalik—the missing link between earlier fossils that had developed an upper arm and an upper thigh (380 MYA) and those with wrist and ankle bones (365 MYA).

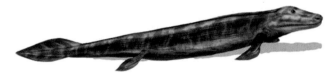

Figure 7.2. *The famous fossil Tiktaalik (the name is Inuit for freshwater fish), which shows a flat head (a change from the conical fish head), a cervical spine, and a distinct upper limb. This fossil is widely hailed as illustrating the successful transition from sea to land.*

While not claiming Tiktaalik to be our direct ancestor, just a distant cousin, Shubin does describe how humans came to develop similar features via our Hox genes, which determine our basic shape and architecture. Slight variations in Hox genes lead to the changes we see in body shape, such as those discovered by Edward Lewis in his manipulation of the genes of the fruit fly (*Drosophila melanogaster*), which produced mutations and rearrangements in body segments. This section of DNA shows very little variation across species throughout the animal kingdom and therefore seems to contain the essential coding for consistent body shape—which explains the general homology noticed by Lovejoy.

It is interesting that whatever mutation led to the development of the upper limb seems to have happened at around the same time as the separation of the head from the thorax via the cervical spine. Before 375 MYA, there was no such thing as a neck, a quite unstable arrangement, especially if it must support 8 percent of the body weight on top of it. This linked evolution of cervical spine and upper limb must therefore be significant, and it should be taken into account when looking at the functional anatomy of the region.

The soft tissues of the shoulder and arms appear to give us the ability to use the weight of the upper girdles to assist the unstable head on top of its perch, while many of our superficial tissues provide a connection between the upper and lower limbs. Both of these arrangements, as might be expected from their recent development, are superficial to the older "core."

■ ARM SWING

There has been much debate on the role of the arms during gait. Everyone seems to accept that there is a contralateral swing with the lower limb, but there is little agreement on the reasons for this. Some believe the swing to be actively driven, while others argue that it is a passive reaction to the rotation created by the legs.

A study by Pontzer, Holloway, Raichlen, and Lieberman (2009) found, as we would expect, that the deltoid is activated during arm swing. What we may not have expected is that each portion of the deltoid contracts in response to the swing—not to create it. Both the anterior and posterior deltoid work eccentrically to decelerate arm swing rather than contracting concentrically to initiate arm movement (fig. 7.3). Because of the deceleration of arm swing, countermovement is once again acting as the stimulus to the muscle fiber, which

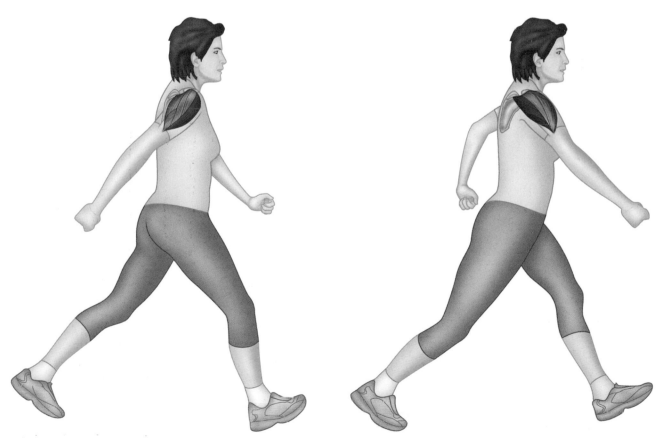

Figure 7.3. The anterior and posterior deltoid respond to the back and forward swing of the arm during gait.

contracts to decelerate the motion and tension the fascial tissue. Pontzer et al. went on to show that much of the movement of the upper limb is a response created by the stride of the legs, and that the upper limb is predominantly acting as a damper of the rotational forces created through the body.

While the study investigated the kinematics of walking (the shape and relationship of the bones) and took EMG readings, it only did so for the deltoid muscle. Measurements were taken with subjects with different levels of arm swing (no swing, normal swing, and weighted swing) when they were running and also when walking. The study showed that arm swing reduced the amount of movement of the head, especially when extra weight was added to the arms. Having no arm swing when running increased upper-body movement by approximately 50 percent, showing that the upper girdle greatly helps to stabilize the head.

Some important conclusions were drawn from the study, as it showed that the damper effect of the arms not only stabilized the head and trunk but also reduced footfall variability. When walking and running with restricted arm swing, there was more variation in step width. Step width may be related to balance, and the fact that it fluctuated when the damper effect of the arms was removed is indicative of the overall balancing role of the shoulder complex, which assists the trunk, the head, and the lower limbs.

The study by Pontzer et al. supports the theories of Harvard paleoanthropologist Daniel Lieberman, who suggests that the low, wide shoulders of *Homo sapiens*, coupled with the strong ligamentum nuchae, assist in reducing the ground reaction forces coming to the head. The ligamentum nuchae (which is formed from the interspinous ligaments and the blending of the trapezius muscles) plays a particularly important role in the damper mechanism.

To my mind, the damper effect is really also a concentration effect—the counterrotation of the shoulder girdle contains the rotation within the trunk and the rotation to the oblique tissues. It therefore adds the stability reported by Pontzer et al. in the form of a reduced variability in footfall, as well as reducing rotational and other forces coming to the head. So far, the effect of arm swing on the efficiency of gait is inconclusive, but that may be because of the small effect it has on calorie use in walking compared to running.

The deltoid can be seen as a continuation of the trapezius, as all of its proximal attachments match those of the distal trapezius, even though any textbook will list them on opposite sides of the clavicle and scapula. This gives the contraction of the deltoid during arm swing a direct connection to the head and the neck ligament, allowing the head to use the energy of the moving arm for stabilization. As Pontzer et al. showed, if you prevent arm swing, the pitch and yaw of the head increases. Lieberman (2011) also shows that the anterior (cleidocranial) portion of the trapezius contracts just prior to heel strike, which links the mass of the arm to the back of the head and helps prevent the head from pitching forward on impact. As he points out, we need this mechanism because the head's center of gravity is in front of the atlanto-occipital joint; extra support behind the axis helps maintain the head's forward gaze (see fig. 7.4).

Chapter 5 showed how the oblique tissues of the abdominals, serratus anterior, rhomboids, and splenii connect the pelvis to the head via the shoulder girdle. The "newer" shoulder musculature of the upper limb, on a separate layer to that of the torso, allows the contralateral rotation between the upper and lower limbs and assists with head stability in the transverse plane. As the rhomboids and the splenii muscles attach through the ligamentum nuchae, they may also tension it, giving further assistance to the trapezius in preventing the forward pitch of the head in the sagittal plane.

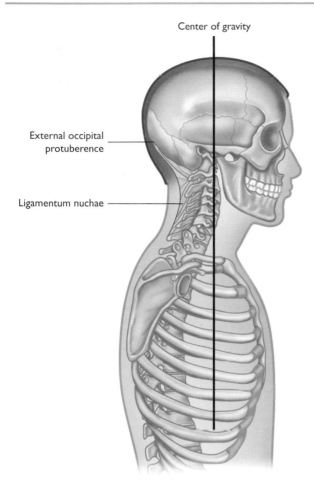

Center of gravity

External occipital
protuberence

Ligamentum nuchae

Figure 7.4. *The ligamentum nuchae is also significant for the support of the head in humans. The skulls of many of our hominid antecessors do not show the tuberosity of the external occipital protuberance. Lieberman hypothesizes that the change in our shoulder girdles, which are wider and lower than those of other hominids, helped develop the ligament, which assists with elastic stability of the head.*

■ CONTRALATERAL SLINGS

Front Functional Line and Anterior Oblique Sling

At the moment of toe-off, the opposite shoulder complex should be at its furthest point from the leg that is toeing off, because of the contralateral arm swing. The pectoralis major and serratus anterior will be contracting slightly to decelerate the backswing of the shoulder complex, and this may allow the arm to create more tension to load the elastic tissue (see figs. 7.5 & 7.6). Two myofascial pathways have been suggested for this relationship:

Myers' "Front Functional Line," with the rectus abdominis from the pectoralis major; and Vleeming's more direct connection from the ribs to the thigh via the "Anterior Oblique Sling" (AOS). The AOS potentially links us from the shoulder girdle (if we add the serratus anterior to the external oblique) to the inside of the opposite thigh via the external to opposite internal obliques and adductors. It is likely, but not yet proven, that both lines may assist efficiency as a result of the contralateral tensioning.

Just as the position of the head can affect recoil in the sagittal plane, as discussed in chapter 3, a similar (though smaller) effect can be felt when the arms either swing out of synch or not at all.

In the research of Pontzer et al. the presence or absence of arm swing made no difference to the metabolic cost of walking. This does not necessarily negate the idea of recoil and its communication through the tissue from the upper body to the lower, since in the research a computer model was used rather than biological tissue. It is possible that the studies done so far have not been sophisticated enough to simultaneously measure elastic loading and other compensatory strategies that the body may employ when one mechanism is taken away.

For example, Pontzer et al. state: "Running may lead to greater stabilizing muscle activity, and therefore a stronger linkage (i.e., a stiffer 'spring') between the pelvis, shoulder, and arm. Stiffer 'springs' may also be necessitated by the greater stride frequencies used in running, since stiffer springs would increase the natural frequencies for the body segments involved."

In other words, the body adapts to the forces acting through it, adjusting the stiffness (when possible) to optimize efficiency. Once again, the myofascia is proving to be self-monitoring, making unconscious calibrations of the soft tissue and using the contractile properties of the muscles as a "stiffness-adjusting system."

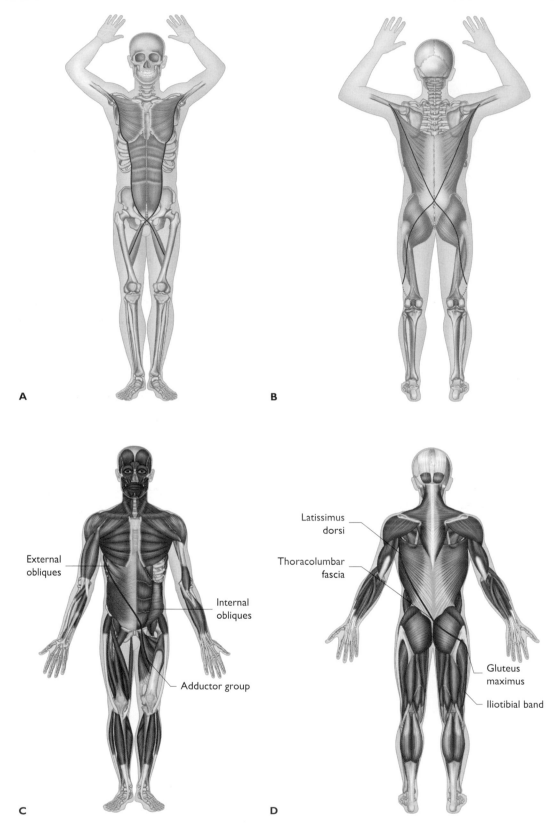

Figure 7.5. *A and B, The Front and Back Functional Lines proposed by Myers. C and D, The Anterior and Posterior Slings proposed by Vleeming.*

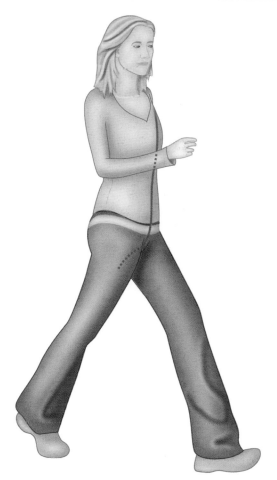

It is obvious that almost all adults can walk with or without arm swing, and while the evidence of its contribution to walking (as opposed to its reaction to the movement) has yet to be found, most walkers have felt the benefits and effects. Our conclusion must be that "more research is necessary" if we want to fully comprehend the downward chain of events from the shoulders.

Back Functional Line and Posterior Oblique Sling

In chapter 5 we saw how the posterior sling is recruited at heel strike to help decelerate pronation: this creates contralateral slings from one humerus to the opposite femur. This relationship has been well investigated by Vleeming and by Zorn. It is worthwhile looking at how the posterior slings interact with the deeper musculature of the back.

Figure 7.6. At toe-off, the Anterior Oblique Sling will be engaged on one side via thoracic extension, hip abduction, and the backswing of the opposite scapula.

By being pre-tensed and contracting in many different directions at heel strike, the lumbar complex can be viewed as an interdependent system (see fig. 7.7). The expansion of one muscle tenses the fascia of another, and

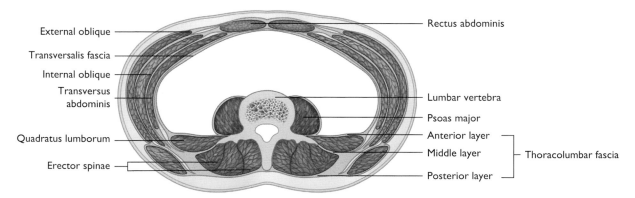

Figure 7.7. At heel strike, the posterior sling will be tensioned across the lower back by hip flexion and opposite arm swing. This pre-tension will assist the deceleration of pronation but will also create a pressure into the erectors. The erectors (especially on the side of the extended leg) will be contracting in their vertical alignment quite strongly and so expanding their volume outward. Both quadrati lumborum will be contracting, dealing with the side flexions and rotations of the transverse processes on both sides. The internal and external obliques and the transversus abdominis will be tensioned by the trunk extension, side flexion, and rotation, and will therefore tension all of the anterior and middle layers of the thoracolumbar fascia. The lower back is a complex arrangement of myofascia contracting and gliding in different directions, and the contraction of each muscle assists the contraction of its neighbors through the hydraulic amplifier effect and parallel pre-tensioning of the tissue.

the lengthening of the fascia created by the position at heel strike will add more power to the contraction. The distribution of fascial tension was investigated by Franklyn-Miller (2009). By performing a straight-leg raise on five cadavers with devices that measured strain at appropriate points, they were able to record the amount of strain created through the leg and lower back (see fig. 7.8).

Iliotibial band	240%
Ipsilateral lumbar fascia	145%
Lateral crural compartment	103%
Achilles tendon	100%
Contralateral lumbar fascia	45%
Plantar fascia	26%

Figure 7.8. *Using strain receptors placed on the listed sections, Franklyn-Miller demonstrated the strain distribution into the myofascial tissue when performing a straight-leg raise. The research was performed on cadavers, showing that the tensioning of the tissue was mechanical and not the result of muscular contraction. The results show the ability of hip flexion to create tension through various tissues, and they also show the wider distribution of that tension—beyond the so-called muscle attachments of the hip extensors.*

Tissue strain occurs at various depths within the body, and each layer needs to move or glide and to facilitate movement beyond the section shown in fig. 7.7. Thankfully, each septum is "lubricated" by the areolar (loose connective) tissue. This tissue is a hydrated and malleable extension of the fascial system, and it allows the layers to glide on one another while maintaining their connection.

Ipsilateral Functional Line

In the second edition of *Anatomy Trains*, Myers added the Ipsilateral Functional Line (IFL), which passes from the lateral aspect of the latissimus dorsi to the external obliques and on to the sartorius. While it is said to be involved in the crawl stroke in swimming, this line may have a more everyday use in its contribution to leg swing after toe-off.

If we look at the lateral tissue at toe-off on the right foot, we see that the right hip and knee are extended and the hip internally rotated, an ideal loading position for the sartorius (see fig. 7.9). The trunk will be relatively side flexed to the opposite side with the arm forward, also ideal for loading the latissimus dorsi and the lateral external obliques.

The resultant elastic loading will be increased by the firing of the external obliques to control the drop of the right ilium, and, once end of range is met, the whole line will then encourage the femur to laterally rotate, the knee and hip to flex (all actions of the sartorius), the right ilium to lift and rotate to the left (external obliques), and finally the shoulder girdle to rotate to the left and the humerus to extend (latissimus dorsi; see figs. 7.10 and 7.11).

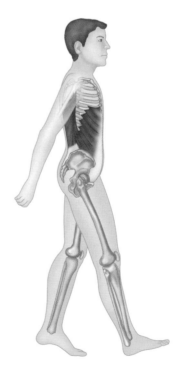

Figure 7.9. *The lateral fibers of the latissimus dorsi will be tensioned by both the arm swing into flexion and the rotation of the shoulder girdle to the opposite side. The almost vertical fibers of the external oblique will be tensioned by the ilium dropping and rotating in the opposite direction from the shoulder girdle.*

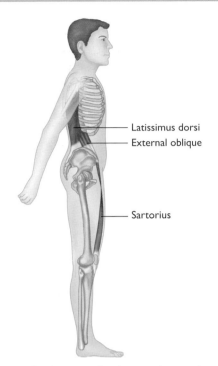

Arm Swing

While the debate on arm swing may be ongoing, we can still use its amplitude and rhythm as an indicator of what may be going on in other regions. Too much swing can be indicative of not enough rotational ability within the trunk, which would make the arms receive more than their normal share. If there is too much swing, check the thoracic rotation ability. If this appears normal, the length of the stride may be too long. It may also be worth investigating other factors: are the arms passive or are they being "driven" to create more swing? If the latter appears to be the case, investigating the historical and/or psychological motivation behind the excessive arm swing may uncover useful insights.

Figure 7.10. Clearly seen in this diagram, the costal attachments of the latissimus dorsi carry into the lateral external obliques, which bring us to the anterior superior iliac spine and the sartorius.

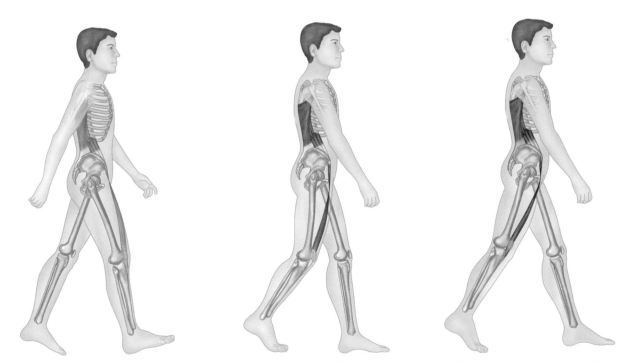

Figure 7.11. With the right Ipsilateral Functional Line naturally shortened because of the hip being flexed, the knee extended, and the shoulder girdle more vertically aligned with the continuity of the latissimus dorsi and external obliques, the leg is more able to "fall" into its loading pattern. With the progression into hip extension during the swing phase and the shoulder girdle recoiling in the opposite direction, we see the gradual tensioning of this line, which can assist with the uncoiling of the leg rotation and can lead to the knee flexion required during the next swing phase.

Front Functional Line and Anterior Oblique Sling

If the arm swing is normal and all of the "essential events" previously mentioned are in place, the Front Functional Line/Anterior Oblique Sling should be able to do its job. The main events for these tissues are hip extension and adduction and thoracic extension, with relative rotation between the pelvis and the thorax, coupled with opposite arm extension.

Back Functional Line and Posterior Oblique Sling

This is almost the exact opposite of the anterior sling. Here, we need hip flexion, posterior tilt of the ilium on the same side, and rotation between the pelvis and the opposite shoulder girdle, coupled with arm flexion.

Ipsilateral Functional Line

For this lateral tissue to engage, the hip and knee must be extended and internally rotated, while the pelvis must be tilted to the same side, and the arm flexed.

▪ SUMMARY

1. The rotational force created by leg swing travels into the torso via the pelvis and is both contained within the torso and lower limb and damped from passing above the shoulders.
2. The trapezius and deltoid help to stabilize the head in the sagittal plane through the ligamentum nuchae.
3. The Front Functional Line/Anterior Oblique Sling uses the humerus and scapula as "anchors" to assist toe-off.
4. The Back Functional Line/Posterior Oblique Sling assists control of the pronation cascade (as discussed in chapter 6) following heel strike.
5. The myofascial complex of the lower back can be seen as an interdependent system using fascial tension and muscle contraction to increase efficiency of the surrounding muscles.
6. All of this system requires the mobility between the layers provided by the loose connective tissue.

8

SPRING WALKER

Did man possess the natural armor of the brutes, he would no longer work as an artificer, nor protect himself with a breast-plate, nor fashion a sword or spear, nor invent a bridle to mount the horse and hunt the lion. Neither could he follow the arts of peace, construct the pipe and the lyre, erect houses, place altars, inscribe laws, and through letters and the ingenuity of the hand hold communion with the wisdom of antiquity, at one time converse with Plato, at another with Aristotle, or Hippocrates.

—Galen

The effectiveness of our bipedal gait has been honed and matured by evolution over the last 4 million years. Walking on two legs was something of a compromise of mobility over stability, because, by standing upright, we put our lower backs and sacroiliac joints at some peril, but the advantages must outweigh these occasional sacrifices.

Coming onto two legs may have decreased our exposure to the sun, and it certainly freed our arms for the control of tools and, eventually, fire. It is metabolically cheaper, allowing us to scavenge further from our home base.

The development of running, and therefore persistence hunting, may have coincided with the capacity for abstract thought—being able to visualize and predict the movement of the hunted animal. Cooking the meat over the fire and sharing thoughts about the hunt (and then embellishing stories about it)—along with the cooperation necessary for the hunt itself—may have helped expand our early language.

All of these factors added to our adaptability and made calories more available to us. We have had larger, stronger, and bigger-brained cousins as ancestors, but we are the ones still around. As the dinosaurs learned—at their cost—bigger is not necessarily better. Our brawnier cousins, the Neanderthals, died out as well. They were sturdier and stronger than *Homo sapiens*, but probably required more calories to survive and presumably were not as agile.

Soft tissues are rarely, if ever, preserved in the fossil record, so we have no way of knowing exactly the difference between our elastic tissue and theirs. But judging from the solidity of Neanderthal bones and those bones' growth patterns and the insertion points, it seems clear that our lighter frame benefits from our fascial system. Our upright stance allows us to load the fascial system through gravity and through forward, backward, lateral, and rotational movement. We benefit from our unstable vertical alignment by letting it challenge and stretch the elastic tissues throughout the body, loading them with energy that we then use for movement, most commonly for walking.

Our survival, however, has been dependent on so much more. With just the minimum tools in terms of muscle power and strength, we have maximized our diversity. While *Homo sapiens* will never outrun a cheetah, lift more weight than a rhino, or swim faster than a dolphin, it is a fact that we can perform all of these activities. No other animal has mastered such a wide range of motion in such a variety of different environments.

Our versatility is unmatched, and we do most motions (once practiced!) with grace, with an ease that is the hallmark of fascial efficiency. As Fukashiro (2006) states, "Most dynamic movements in sports activities involve a countermovement, where an agonist muscle contracts after being stretched in an eccentric phase, which is usually defined as a stretch shortening cycle." Essentially, by going in the direction opposite to the one we want to travel in, we are using the efficient dynamics of the stretch-shortening cycle, which is "the natural way of muscle function in normal locomotion … nature's way to combine the available resources … in such a way that both peak performance and movement economy are considered in the most appropriate way in each particular movement situation" (Komi 2011).

When we match joint alignment with the pull of gravity and the ground reaction force— coupled with the momentum involved in any movement—we can see how the dynamics are channeled into the elastic tissues. By exploiting the instability of our vertical alignment and smooth joints, we easily gain countermovement. The mechanoreceptors embedded within our wonderful three-dimensional web of fascial tissue activate the necessary muscles to decelerate the action that stretches the elastic fascial tissue, which can assist the recovery movement with metabolically "free" energy.

When we look at Muybridge's horse progressing from a trot to a gallop, we see increases in flexion and extension, the greater movement putting more load into the tissues to support and produce the stronger forces required. The quadruped is more clearly a full-body walker; the quote that began this book shows that we have yet to appreciate the full involvement of our anatomy in locomotion, since half of it is sadly labeled the "passenger" (Perry and Burnfield 2010).

I think it is an interesting exercise to take the two transition points—heel strike and toe-off— and reverse engineer them by simply looking at where the forces are traveling. At toe-off, we have progressed our pelvis forward from the back foot to create a line of tension along the entire front of the body (Figs. 8.1–8.9).

If we look back to the work of Huijing, mentioned in chapter 1, in which he examined the transfer of force from one tendon into the

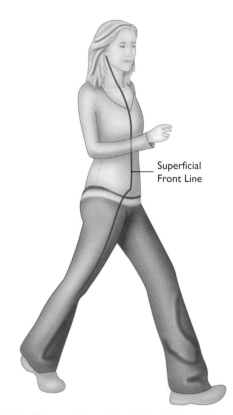

Superficial Front Line

Figure 8.1.　The continuity of the SFL is challenged but the toe-off position strains much of the anterior tissues, especially the vertically aligned muscle fibers. By going into extension, we have put kinetic energy into many of the flexors, to be released at toe-off.

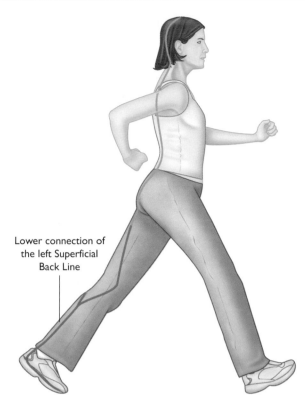

Lower connection of the left Superficial Back Line

Figure 8.2. At toe off, the toe extension and knee extension have strained the lower leg.

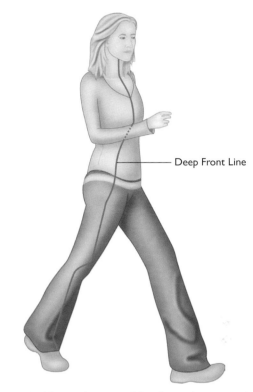

Deep Front Line

Figure 8.4. The combination of dorsiflexion, knee extension, hip extension, abduction, and internal rotation is the ideal position to lengthen the Deep Front Line, which will assist with almost all the required events at toe-off.

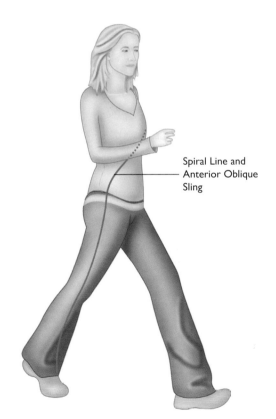

Spiral Line and Anterior Oblique Sling

Figure 8.3. The counterrotation of the shoulder girdle creates the tension through the oblique tissues.

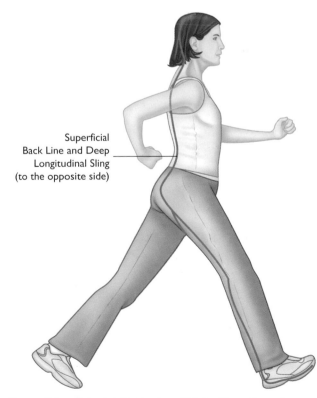

Superficial Back Line and Deep Longitudinal Sling (to the opposite side)

Figure 8.5. At heel strike, the flexed hip position will require support from all of the hip extensors. They will be in a pre-tensioned position because of the flexion, and Vleeming's Deep Longitudinal Sling may assist with sacroiliac stability after heel strike.

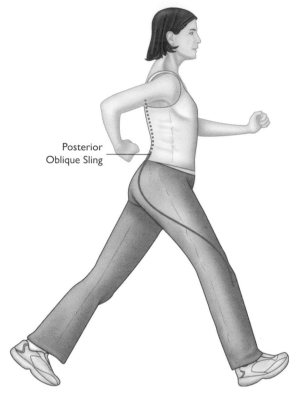

Figure 8.6. *At heel strike, we can follow the rotational forces caused by the tilt of the calcaneus to bring us to the superior portion of the gluteus maximus from the tibialis anterior and the ITB. From there, we carry into the latissimus dorsi to create a form of sling (as used by Zorn and Vleeming). This superficial sling addresses the rotational aspects of the pronation pattern, while the Deep Longitudinal Sling helps balance the sacroiliac joint through the connection to the sacrotuberous ligament and the long dorsal sacroiliac ligament on the opposite side.*

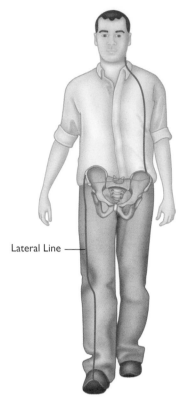

Figure 8.7. *With the center of gravity at the midline of the body offset from the point of support, the hip is encouraged into adduction on the side of heel strike, which loads the hip abductors on that side. Meanwhile, the hip adductors, lateral abdominals, and quadratus lumborum must open on the opposite side.*

surrounding tissue, we can now really appreciate the complexity and beauty of the myofascial arrangements. Working as a separator, connector, force concentrator, force damper, and force-dispersal system, the myofascial system not only communicates mechanical information directly through its fibers but also senses and adjusts the sectional stiffness according to the forces acting at any one time.

■ FOOTWEAR

Nature, Mr. Allnut, is what we are put in this world to rise above.

—Rose Sayer (played by Katharine Hepburn) in *The African Queen*

One of the most obvious ways we try to rise above nature is through adornment, and, when not passing our time inventing new methods of maiming and killing each other, humanity has often diverted its attention to novel ways of mutilating the body we inherited. From foot binding to winklepickers, stilettos to platform boots, each generation and each culture has managed to find a way to interfere with the natural dynamics of our feet. When left to their own devices, our feet serve us quite well, and they really need little more than some protective covering to save us from the vagaries of litter and sharp (or sometimes squidgy) objects.

Hopefully by this stage of the book, enough evidence of the interaction between anatomy, function, and evolution has been presented to convince you of their interrelationship.

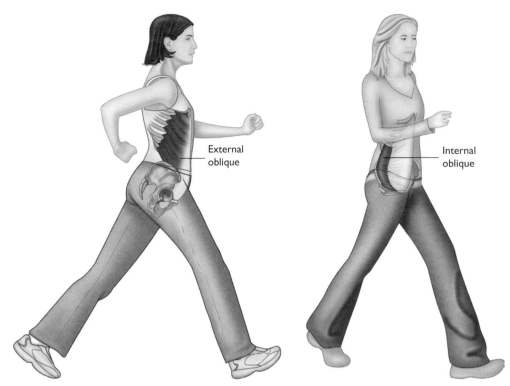

Figure 8.8. *With the pelvis moving further and faster than the rib cage, the Xs of the lateral abdominals will be stretched in opposite directions on each side. These "ipsilateral" obliques therefore carry the rotation created by bipedal gait into the intercostals—this is damped by the counterrotation of the arms and the "contralateral" obliques (see fig. 8.3).*

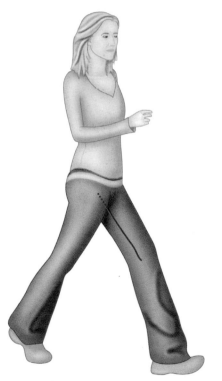

Figure 8.9. *As the leg swings through into hip flexion, the adductor magnus on the swing leg will be lengthened, in order to pre-tension it prior to heel strike, when it will work to resist further flexion. During the swing phase, it may help to tension the deep posterior compartment fascia to supinate the foot prior to heel strike.*

So, with apologies to Miss Sayer, we would be better served by not trying to rise above our nature, at least in the foot department. A thick sole will dampen our proprioceptive feedback (Saxby 2011). An elevated heel will force more of the body weight onto the metatarsal heads, stressing them, and it will shorten the Achilles tendon, distorting the posture and interfering with the communication through the lines. An elevation of two inches will give the body an incline of 20 degrees, leading to a 23 percent increase in the load on the front of the knees. A three-inch heel puts 76 percent of the body weight on the metatarsal heads, which are not designed for that kind of constant stress (see fig. 8.10).

Cramped toe boxes lead to misalignment of the first and fifth toes (predominantly, though in many cases the others can be affected as well), which leads to varied angles at toe-off (see fig. 8.11). This can be further exacerbated by the longitudinal axis of the shoe, which is often curved, especially in athletic shoes.

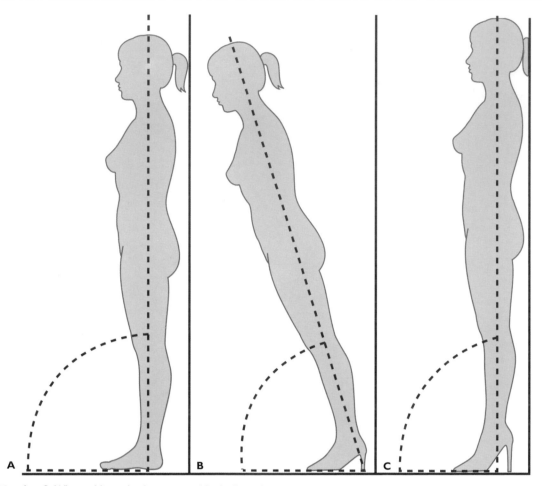

Figure 8.10. *A to B, When adding a heel to a neutral body, the incline created by the heel has to be compensated for somewhere in the body: at the knee, the hips, the lumbar spine, or the thoracic spine, depending on one's tendency. This places undue stress on any or all of those areas, increasing the likelihood of pain and dysfunction. C, As the heel increases in height, an ever-greater percentage of body weight is brought to the ball of the foot, decreasing efficiency and increasing stress on the bones. (Adapted from Dalton 2011.)*

A shoe is not only a design, but it's a part of your body language, the way you walk. The way you're going to move is quite dictated by your shoes.

—Christian Louboutin

For a normal foot, the ideal shoe would be flat (see fig. 8.11B). Wearing a minimal sole allows clear proprioception, but it should be thick enough and strong enough to offer protection. A wider toe box gives the toes room to spread on contact with the ground, which is mechanically useful. As the metatarsals spread, the interossei will be stretched, signaling a reflex contraction of the quadriceps (Michaud 2011). A simple arrangement of the shoe, one in which the alignment of the foot is unaltered, is ideal. It will allow the joints to work through their normal range, loading the appropriate tissue through the progression from heel strike to toe-off.

Anything that interferes with joint alignment will affect our ability to use the longer springs of the body. Wearing high heels not only places more weight on the metatarsal heads but also prevents the ankle from dorsiflexing, while cramped or angled toe boxes will force toe-off to occur at angles other than the ideal first and second metatarsal heads.

Various "fitness" and "technology" shoes have appeared on the market over the last ten years—many making health and beauty claims.

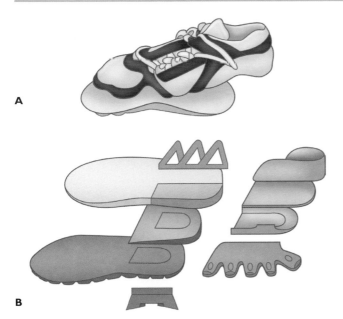

Figure 8.11. *The "normal" shoe (A) has many supposedly positive features. Running shoes, in particular, may include "motion control," extra heel cushioning, and a curved longitudinal axis. Some of these features may be necessary for challenged feet, but they will interfere with the natural architecture and function. Thicker soles dampen proprioception; motion control, strangely enough, prevents motion, which also lessens proprioception communication through the body and inhibits some of the normal tissue responses described in this book. The cramped and angled toe box will affect the foot's ability to spread and then push off at an optimal angle. A minimal shoe (B) simply provides protection from the elements and unseen objects. The thin and pliable sole allows the foot to feel the ground and make appropriate responses, while the wide toe box and lack of curving from heel to toe facilitate actions of the metatarsals, from the spreading at heel strike to the correct angle at toe-off.*

One of the reasons why they claim to "help you lose weight," "burn more calories," or "give you long lean legs" is the fact that they alter the body's natural mechanics. We have evolved to make walking as easy and as calorie efficient as possible, so by interfering with that process, we have to compensate with muscle work. When we do so, however, we are also at threat of changing the forces that flow through the joints, making these "technology" shoes unsuitable for many people, if any.

> **Most shoes are shaped as if feet were made for shoes.**
>
> —Mokokoma Mokhonoana

Many people, because of inherited characteristics, accidents, or misuse, no longer have the ideal alignment through the joints of the feet. They may benefit from the use of orthotics to retain efficiency. I believe orthotics to be an intervention of last resort, preferring to use manual therapy, manipulation, and/or exercise to normalize the foot as much as possible. If orthotics are to be used, they should be expertly fitted, and the client should be monitored by an experienced clinician to assess the rest of the body's adaptation to the orthotics. Too often, orthopedic insoles are prescribed, and then the job is considered done. The body will require time, however—and possibly some assistance—to recognize the new position it is in, and so a full screening of the "essential events" should be repeated.

> **I have two doctors, my left leg and my right.**
>
> —G. M. Trevelyan

> **But the beauty is in the walking—we are betrayed by destinations.**
>
> —Gwyn Thomas

9

CONCLUSION

Whether you believe our form has been honed over 4 billion years of evolution or designed by some greater force, I hope this text has given you tools for a deeper appreciation of how its parts mingle and amalgamate. Our vertical alignment, our joint arrangement, and our soft-tissue properties work together in a cooperative pact to provide us with new and efficient movement possibilities. The cumulative changes over time have honed our system to use fewer calories for walking, presumably so that they can be redirected to support our increased brain size.

Efficiency is enhanced by many aspects of our myofascial system, which can capture kinetic energy as strain and reuse it in a return movement. Tissue strain is caused by momentum and the various offsets of gravity and ground reaction force acting through our skeletal system. The skeletal joints direct the forces into the soft tissue, where we try to minimize the lengthening or shortening of muscle fibers.

When the walking system is working correctly—joints are aligned, tissues are healthy, and momentum is maintained—the experience can be one of joy and ease. Any deviation from that ideal means that something has to work harder. I believe that one of the

keys to our success as a species has been our adaptability under stress. Our systems can find alternative strategies for success—we are bioplastic. No matter if is a loss of brain function or the loss of a limb, we are able to find new pathways to our goals.

One of the main fallback strategies for movement is to use concentric and eccentric contractions—to do extra work in order to make up for the loss of momentum or the loss of tissue strain, or to deal with strain going in the wrong direction. Whether or not any of these changes causes pathology is up for debate in other forums, but pathologies will certainly influence our efficiency.

The purpose of the essential events is to provide a way of searching through the complexities of a "walking system" to seek out where there might be energy leakages. By working to renew the range in a joint or tissue, bringing better alignment between joints and forces, I hope that one can also bring better alignment and increased communication to a client, a friend, or a relative. It is my greatest hope that small changes for them will assist their experience of their bodies, and that they will feel the connection within themselves and to everything else around them.

Walking in the mountain with bare foot,
Teasing the flowers with heavy soot,
Touching the grasses, climbing the
horses, swinging the girls
It is joyful, jolly like the flying.
Swimming in the rivers, tearing the
clothes and burning the shoes
Angel of the nature; counting the
grasses, touching the flower, teasing
the birds

—M. F. Moonzajer, *LOVE, HATRED AND MADNESS*

BIBLIOGRAPHY

Compiled with thanks to Robert Miller.

Abitbol, M. 1988. "Effect of Posture and Locomotion on Energy Expenditure." *American Journal of Physical Anthropology* 77 (2): 191–199.

Aiello, L., and C. Dean. 2002. *An Introduction to Human Evolutionary Anatomy*. London: Academic Press.

Arampatzis, A., A. Peper, S. Bierbaum, and K. Albracht. 2010. "Plasticity of Human Achilles Tendon Mechanical and Morphological Properties in Response to Cyclic Strain." *Journal of Biomechanics* 43 (16): 3073–3079.

Arampatzis, A., S. Stafilidis, G. DeMonte, K. Karamanidis, G. Morey-Klapsing, and G. P. Brüggemann. 2005. "Strain and Elongation of the Human Gastrocnemius Tendon and Aponeurosis during Maximal Plantar flexion Effort." *Journal of Biomechanics* 38 (4): 833–841.

Ardrey, R. 1961. *African Genesis: A Personal Investigation into the Animal Origins and Nature of Man*. London: Collins.

Baker, R., R. Souza, and M. Fredericson. 2011. "Iliotibial Band Syndrome: Soft Tissue and Biomechanical Factors in Evaluation and Treatment." *PM&R* 3 (6): 550–561.

Beach, P. 2010. *Muscles and Meridians: The Manipulation of Shape*. Edinburgh, UK: Churchill Livingstone Elsevier.

Bell, C. 1837. *The Hand: Its Mechanism and Vital Endowments as Evincing Design*. London: William Pickering.

Biewener, A. A. 1998. "Muscle-Tendon Stresses and Elastic Energy Storage during Locomotion in the Horse." *Comparative Biochemistry and Physiology: Part B, Biochemistry and Molecular Biology* 120 (1): 73–87.

Biewener, A. 2016. "Locomotion as an Emergent Property of Muscle Contractile Dynamics." *Journal of Experimental Biology* 219 (2): 285–294.

Blazevich, A. 2011. "The Stretch-Shortening Cycle." In Cardinale, Newton, and Nosaka 2011, 209–222.

Böl, M., H. Stark, and N. Schilling. 2011. "On a Phenomenological Model for Fatigue Effects in Skeletal Muscles." *Journal of Theoretical Biology* 281 (1): 122–132.

Bourke, J. 2011. *What It Means to Be Human: Reflections from 1791 to the Present*. London: Virago.

Bramble, D. M., and D. E. Lieberman. 2004. "Endurance Running and the Evolution of *Homo*." *Nature* 432: 345–352.

Calais-Germain, B. 1993. *Anatomy of Movement*. Seattle, WA: Eastland Press.

Cardinale, M., R. Newton, and K. Nosaka, eds. 2011. *Strength and Conditioning: Biological Principles and Practical Applications*. Oxford: Wiley-Blackwell.

Carmont, M. R., A. M. Highland, J. R. Rochester, E. M. Paling, and M. B. Davies. 2011. "An Anatomical and Radiological Study of the Fascia Cruris and Paratenon of the Achilles Tendon." *Foot and Ankle Surgery* 17 (3): 186–192.

Cochran, G., and H. Harpending. 2010. *The 10,000 Year Explosion: How Civilization Accelerated Human Evolution.* New York: Basic Books.

Conroy, G., and H. Pontzer. 2012. *Reconstructing Human Origins.* New York: W. W. Norton.

Crompton, R., E. Vereecke, and S. Thorpe. 2008. "Locomotion and Posture From the Common Hominoid Ancestor To Fully Modern Hominins, With Special Reference to the Last Common Panin/Hominin Ancestor." *Journal of Anatomy* 212 (4): 501–543.

Dalton, E., ed. 2011. *Dynamic Body: Exploring Form Expanding Function.* Oklahoma City: Freedom from Pain Institute.

Dalton, E., M. Bishop, M. D. Tillman, and C. J. Hass. 2011. "Simple Change in Standing Position Enhances the Initiation of Gait." *Medicine and Science in Sports and Exercise* 43 (12): 2352–2358.

Dart, R. 1996. *Alexander Center.* www.alexandercenter.com/dartspirals.html.

Darwin, C. 1874. *Descent of Man.* London: John Murray.

DeRosa, C., and J. A. Porterfield. 2007. "Anatomical Linkages and Muscle Slings of the Lumbopelvic Region." In Vleeming, Mooney, and Stoeckart 2007, 47–62.

DeSilva, J. 2010. "Revisiting the 'Midtarsal Break.'" *American Journal of Physical Anthropology* 141: 245–258.

Doral, M. N., M. Alam, M. Bozkurt, E. Turhan, O. A. Atay, G. Dönmez, and N. Maffulli. 2010. "Functional Anatomy of the Achilles Tendon." *Knee Surgery, Sports Traumatology, Arthroscopy* 18 (5): 638–643.

Earls, J. 2014. *Born to Walk,* 1st edn. Berkeley, CA: North Atlantic Books.

Earls, J., and T. Myers. 2010. *Fascial Release for Structural Balance.* Berkeley, CA: North Atlantic Books.

Fernández, P., S. Almécija, B. Patel, C. Orr, M. Tocheri, and W. Jungers. 2015. "Functional Aspects of Metatarsal Head Shape in Humans, Apes, and Old World Monkeys." *Journal of Human Evolution* 86: 136–146.

Filler, A. G. 2007. *The Upright Ape: A New Origin of the Species.* Franklin Lakes, NJ: Career Press.

Franklyn-Miller, A., E. Falvey, R. Clark, A. Bryant, P. Brukner, P. Barker, C. Briggs, and P. McCrory. 2009. "The Strain Patterns of the Deep Fascia of the Lower Limb." In Huijing, Hollander, Findley, and Schleip 2009, 150–151.

Fukashiro, S., D. C. Hay, and A. Nagano. 2006. "Biomechanical Behavior of Muscle-Tendon Complex during Dynamic Human Movements." *Journal of Applied Biomechanics* 22 (2): 131–147.

Fukunaga, T., Y. Kawakami, K. Kubo, and H. Kanehisa. 2002. "Muscle and Tendon Interaction during Human Movements." *Exercise and Sport Sciences Reviews* 30 (3): 106–110.

Gracovetsky, S. 2008. *The Spinal Engine.* Montreal: Serge Gracovetsky, PhD.

Hawks, J. 2009. "How Strong Is a Chimpanzee, Really?" *Slate.* February 25. www.slate.com/articles/health_and_science/science/2009/02/how_strong_is_a_chimpanzee.html.

Heinrich, B. 2002. *Why We Run: A Natural History.* New York: Ecco.

Hewett, T., T. Lynch, G. Myer, K. Ford, R. Gwin, and R. Heidt. 2009. "Multiple Risk Factors Related to Familial Predisposition to Anterior Cruciate Ligament Injury: Fraternal Twin Sisters with Anterior Cruciate Ligament Ruptures." *British Journal of Sports Medicine* 44 (12): 848–855.

Hodges, P. W., and K. Tucker. 2011. "Moving Differently in Pain: A New Theory to Explain the Adaptation to Pain." *Pain* 152: S90–S98.

Holowka, N., and D. Lieberman. 2018. "Rethinking the Evolution of the Human Foot: Insights from Experimental Research." *Journal of Experimental Biology* 221 (17): jeb174425.

Hoyt, D., and C. Taylor. 1981. "Gait and the Energetics of Locomotion in Horses." *Nature* 292 (5820): 239–240.

Huijing, P. A. 1999a. "Muscle as a Collagen Fiber Reinforced Composite Material: Force Transmission in Muscle and Whole Limbs." *Journal of Biomechanics* 32 (4): 329–345.

———. 1999b. "Muscular Force Transmission: A Unified, Dual or Multiple System? A Review and Some Explorative Experimental Results." *Archives of Physiology and Biochemistry* 170 (4): 292–311.

———. 2009. "Epimuscular Myofascial Force Transmission: A Historical Perspective and Implications for New Research." *Journal of Biomechanics* 42: 9–21.

Huijing, P., and G. Baan. 2008. "Myofascial Force Transmission via Extramuscular Pathways Occurs between Antagonistic Muscles." *Cells, Tissues, Organs* 188 (4): 400–414.

Huijing, P. A., A. Yaman, C. Ozturk, and C. A. Yucesoy. 2011. "Effects Angle on Global and Local Strains within Human Triceps Surae Muscle: MRI Analysis Indicating In Vivo Myofascial Force Transmission between Synergistic Muscles." *Surgical and Radiological Anatomy* 33 (10): 869–879.

Huijing, P. A., P. Hollander, T. W. Findley, and R. Schliep, eds. 2009. *Fascia Research II: Basic Science and Implications for Conventional and Complementary Health Care*. Edinburgh, UK: Elsevier.

Ingber, D. 1998. "The Architecture of Life." *Scientific American* 278 (1): 48–57.

Ingold, T. 2004. "Culture on the Ground: The World Perceived through the Feet." *Journal of Material Culture* 9 (3): 315–340.

Inwood, S. 2003. *The Forgotten Genius: The Biography of Robert Hooke, 1635–1703*. San Francisco: MacAdam/Cage.

Ireland, M. L., J. D. Willson, B. T. Ballantyne, and I. McClay Davis. 2003. "Hip Strength in Females with and without Patellofemoral Pain." *Journal of Orthopaedic & Sports Physical Therapy* 33 (11): 671–676.

Jaspers, R. T., R. Brunner, U. N. Riede, and P. A. Huijing. 2005. "Healing of the Aponeurosis during Recovery from Aponeurotomy: Morphological and Histological Adaptation and Related Changes in Mechanical Properties." *Journal of Orthopaedic Research* 23 (2): 266–273.

Jielile, J., J. P. Bai, G. Sabirhazi, D. Redat, T. Yilihamu, B. Xinlin, G. Hu, B. Tang, B. Liang, and Q. Sun. 2010. "Factors Influencing the Tensile Strength of Repaired Achilles Tendon: A Biomechanical Experiment Study." *Clinical Biomechanics* 25 (8): 789–795.

Kawakami, Y., T. Muraoka, S. Ito, H. Kanehisa, and T. Fukunaga. 2002. "In Vivo Muscle Fibre Behaviour during Counter-movement Exercise in Humans Reveals a Significant Role for Tendon Elasticity." *Journal of Physiology* 540 (2): 635–646.

Kawakami, Y., N. Sugisaki, K. Chino, and T. Fukunaga. 2006. "Tendon Mechanical Properties: Influence of Muscle Actions." *Journal of Biomechanics* 39: S65.

Kendall, F. P., E. K. McCreary, P. G. Provance, M. M. Rodgers, and W. A. Romani. 2005. *Muscles: Testing and Function with Posture and Pain*. Baltimore, MD: Lippincott, Williams and Wilkins.

Kjaer, M. 2004. "Role of Extracellular Matrix in Adaptation of Tendon and Skeletal Muscle to Mechanical Loading." *Physiological Reviews* 84 (2): 649–698.

Kjaer, M., H. Langberg, K. Heinemeier, M. L. Bayer, M. Hansen, L. Holm, S. Doessing, M. Kongsgaard, M. R. Krogsgaard, and S. P. Magnusson. 2009. "From Mechanical Loading to Collagen Synthesis, Structural Changes and Function in Human Tendon." *Scandinavian Journal of Medicine and Science in Sports* 19 (4): 500–510.

Komi, P., ed. 2011. *Neuromuscular Aspects of Sport Performance*. Chichester, UK: Blackwell.

Kongsgaard, M., C. H. Nielson, S. Hegnsvad, P. Aagaard, and S. P. Magnusson. 2011. "Mechanical Properties of the Human Achilles Tendon, In Vivo." *Clinical Biomechanics* 26 (7): 772–777.

Latash, M. L. 2012. *Fundamentals of Motor Control*. Waltham, MA: Academic Press.

Levin, S. M. 2007. "A Suspensory System for the Sacrum in Pelvic Mechanics: Biotensegrity." In Vleeming, Mooney, and Stoeckart 2007, 229–238.

Lichtwark, G. A., and A. M. Wilson. 2007. "Is Achilles Tendon Compliance Optimised for Maximum Muscle Efficiency during Locomotion?" *Journal of Biomechanics* 40 (8): 1768–1775.

Lieberman, D. 2011. *The Evolution of the Human Head*. Cambridge, MA: Belknap Press of Harvard University Press.

Lieberman, D. 2012. "Those Feet in Ancient Times." *Nature* 483 (7391): 550–551.

Lovejoy, C. O. 2007. "Evolution of the Human Lumbopelvic Region and Its Relationship to Some Clinical Deficits of the Spine and Pelvis." In Vleeming, Mooney, and Stoeckart 2007, 141–158.

Maloiy G. M., N. C. Heglund, L. M. Prager, G. A. Cavagna, and C. R. Taylor. 1986. "Energetic Cost of Carrying Loads: Have African Women Discovered an Economic Way?" *Nature* 319: 668–669.

Malvankar, S., and Khan, W. S. 2011. "Evolution of the Achilles Tendon: The Athlete's Achilles Heel?" *Foot* 21 (4): 193–197.

Maus, H. M., S. W. Lipfert, M. Gross, J. Rummel, and A. Seyfarth. 2010. "Upright Human Gait Did Not Provide a Major Mechanical Challenge for Our Ancestors." *Nature Communications* September 7.

McArdle, W. D. 2010. *Exercise Physiology: Nutrition, Energy and Human Performance*. New York: Lippincott, Williams and Wilkins.

McCredie, S. 2007. *Balance: In Search of the Lost Sense*. New York: Little, Brown.

McDougall, C. 2010. *Born to Run: The Hidden Tribe, the Ultra-runners and the Greatest Race the World Has Never Seen*. London: Profile Books.

McKeon, P., J. Hertel, D. Bramble, and I. Davis. 2014. "The Foot Core System: A New Paradigm for Understanding Intrinsic Foot Muscle Function." *British Journal of Sports Medicine* 49 (5): 290.

McNeill Alexander, R. 1986. "Human Energetics: Making Headway in Africa." *Nature* 319: 623–624.

———. 1992. *The Human Machine: How the Body Works*. London: Natural History Museum.

———. 1995. "Elasticity in Mammalian Backs." Second Interdisciplinary World Conference on Low Back Pain: The Integrated Function of the Lumbar Spine and Sacroiliac Joints.

———. 2002. "Tendon Elasticity and Muscle Function." *Comparative Biochemistry and Physiology Part A: Molecular & Integrative Physiology* 133 (4): 1001–1011.

———. 2005. *Energy for Animal Life*. Oxford: Oxford University Press.

———. 2006. *Principles of Animal Locomotion*. Princeton, NJ: Princeton University Press.

Meredith, M. 2011. *Born in Africa: The Quest for the Origins of Human Life*. London: Simon and Schuster.

Michaud, T. 2011. *Human Locomotion: The Conservative Management of Gait-Related Disorders*. Newton, MA: Newton Biomechanics.

Middleditch, A., and J. Oliver. 2005. *Functional Anatomy of the Spine*. Edinburgh, UK: Elsevier.

Morgan, E. 1990. *The Scars of Evolution: What Our Bodies Tell Us about Human Origins*. Worcester, UK: Billing and Sons.

Morton, D. J. 1952. *Human Locomotion and Body Form: A Study of Gravity and Man*. Baltimore, MD: Williams and Wilkins.

Muller, D., and R. Schleip. 2011. "Fascial Fitness: Fascia Oriented Training for Bodywork and Movement Therapies." *Terra Rosa* 7: 2–11. www.terrarosa.com.au/articles/Terra_News7.pdf.

Muscolino, J. 2006. *Kinesiology: The Skeletal System and Muscle Function*. St. Louis, MO: Mosby.

Myers, T. W. 2001, 2009, 2015. *Anatomy Trains: Myofascial Meridians for Manual and Movement Therapists*, 1st, 2nd, 3rd edns. Edinburgh, UK: Churchill Livingstone Elsevier.

Nene, A., C. Byrne, and H. Hermens. 2004. "Is Rectus Femoris Really a Part of Quadriceps?", *Gait & Posture* 20 (1): 1–13.

Nicholson, G. 2009. *The Lost Art of Walking: The History, Science, Philosophy, and Literature of Pedestrianism*. New York: Riverhead Books.

O'Keefe, J. H., R. Vogel, C. J. Lavie, and L. Cordain. 2011. "Exercise Like a Hunter-Gatherer: A Prescription for Organic Physical Fitness." *Progress in Cardiovascular Diseases* 53 (6): 471–479.

Olsen, B. D. 2009. *Understanding Human Anatomy through Evolution*. Morrisville, NC: Lulu Press.

Ortega, J. D., and C. T. Farley. 2005. "Minimizing Center of Mass Vertical Movement Increases Metabolic Cost in Walking." *Journal of Applied Physiology* 99 (6): 2099–2107.

Osborn, H. 1928. "The Influence of Bodily Locomotion in Separating Man from the Monkeys and Apes." *The Scientific Monthly* May: 385–399.

Oschman, J. 2003. *Energy Medicine in Therapeutics and Human Performance*. Edinburgh, UK: Butterworth Heinemann.

Parker, P. J., and C. A. Briggs. 2007. "Anatomy and Biomechanics of the Lumbar Fasciae: Implications for Lumbopelvic Control and Clinical Practice." In Vleeming, Mooney, and Stoeckart 2007, 63–74.

Perry, J., and J. M. Burnfield. 2010. *Gait Analysis*. Thorofare, NJ: Slack.

Pichler, W., N. P. Tesch, W. Grechenig, O. Leithgoeb, and G. Windisch. 2007. "Anatomic Variations of the Musculotendinous Junction of the Soleus Muscle and Its Clinical Implications." *Clinical Anatomy* 20 (4): 444–447.

Pontzer, H. 2017. "Economy and Endurance in Human Evolution." *Current Biology* 27 (12): R613–21.

Pontzer, H., J. H. Holloway, D. A. Raichlen, and D. E. Lieberman. 2009. "Control and Function of Arm Swing in Human Walking and Running." *Journal of Experimental Biology* 212 (6): 894.

Powers, C. M. n.d. *Biomechanical Factors Contributing to Patellofemoral Pain; The Dynamic QAngle*. Musculoskeletal Biomechanics Research Lab, University of Southern California.

———. n.d. *Dynamic Stabilization of the Patellofemoral Joint: Stabilization from Above and Below*. Musculoskeletal Biomechanics Research Lab, University of Southern California.

———. 2003. "The Influence of Altered Lower-Extremity Kinematics on Patellofemoral Joint Dysfunction: A Theoretical Perspective." *Journal of Orthopaedic & Sports Physical Therapy* 33 (11): 639–646.

———. 2010. "The Influence of Abnormal Hip Mechanics on Knee Injury: A Biomechanical Perspective." *Journal of Orthopaedic & Sports Physical Therapy* 40 (2): 42–51.

Powers, C. M., S. R. Ward, M. Fredericson, M. Guillet, and F. G. Shellock. 2003. "Patellofemoral Kinematics during Weight-bearing and Non-weight-bearing Knee Extension in Persons with Lateral Subluxation of the Patella: A Preliminary Study." *Journal of Orthopaedic & Sports Physical Therapy* 33 (11): 677–685.

Premkumar, K. 2004. *The Massage Connection: Anatomy and Physiology*. Baltimore, MD: Lippincott, Williams and Wilkins.

Richards, J. 2008. *Biomechanics in Clinic and Research*. Edinburgh, UK: Churchill Livingstone Elsevier.

Roberts, T. 2016. "Contribution of Elastic Tissues to the Mechanics and Energetics of Muscle Function during Movement." *Journal of Experimental Biology* 219 (2): 266–275.

Roberts, T., and E. Azizi. 2011. "Flexible Mechanisms: The Diverse Roles of Biological Springs in Vertebrate Movement." *Journal of Experimental Biology* 214 (3): 353–361.

Rolf, I., and R. Feitis. 1991. *Rolfing and physical reality*. Healing Arts Press.

Rubenson, J., N. Pires, H. Loi, G. Pinniger, and D. Shannon. 2012. "On the Ascent: The Soleus Operating Length is Conserved to the Ascending Limb of the Force-Length Curve Across Gait Mechanics in Humans." *Journal of Experimental Biology* 215 (20): 3539–3551.

Sahrmann, S. A. 2002. *Diagnosis and Treatment of Movement Impairment Syndromes*. St. Louis, MO: Mosby.

Sawicki, G., C. Lewis, and D. Ferris. 2009. "It Pays to Have a Spring in Your Step." *Exercise and Sport Sciences Reviews* 37 (3): 130–138.

Saxby, L. 2011. *Proprioception: Making Sense of Barefoot Running*. London: Terra Plana International.

Schleip, R., and A. Baker, eds, 2015. *Fascia in Sport and Movement*, 1st edn. Edinburgh: Handspring.

Schleip, R., T. W. Findley, L. Chaitow, and P. Huijing. 2012. *Fascia: The Tensional Network of the Human Body*. Edinburgh, UK: Churchill Livingstone Elsevier.

Shih, Y., Y. Chen, Y. Lee, M. Chan, and T. Shiang. 2016. "Walking Beyond Preferred Transition Speed Increases Muscle Activations with a Shift from Inverted Pendulum to Spring Mass Model in Lower Extremity." *Gait & Posture* 46: 5–10.

Shubin, N. 2008. *Your Inner Fish: A Journey into the 3.5-billion-year History of the Human Body*. London: Allen Lane.

Silder, A., B. Whittington, B. Heiderscheit, and D. Thelen. 2007. "Identification of Passive Elastic Joint Moment–Angle Relationships in the Lower Extremity." *Journal of Biomechanics* 40 (12): 2628–2635.

Solnit, R. 2002. *Wanderlust: A History of Walking*. London: Verso.

Spoor, F., Hublin, J., Braun, M., and Zonneveld, F. 2003. "The bony labyrinth of Neanderthals." *Journal of Human Evolution*, 44 (2): 141–165.

Stringer, C. 2011. *The Origin of Our Species*. London: Allen Lane.

Stringer, C., and P. Andrews. 2011. *The Complete World of Human Evolution*. London: Thames and Hudson.

Tattersall, I. 2007. *Becoming Human: Evolution and Human Uniqueness*. Oxford: Oxford University Press.

Thompson, D. 1940. *Science and the Classics, by D'Arcy W. Thompson*. London: H. Milford.

Tudge, C., and J. Young. 2009. *The Link: Uncovering Our Earliest Ancestors*. London: Little, Brown.

van Wingerden, J., A. Vleeming, C. Snijders, and R. Stoeckart. 1993. "A Functional-Anatomical Approach to the Spine-Pelvis Mechanism: Interaction between the Biceps Femoris Muscle and the Sacrotuberous Ligament." *European Spine Journal* 2 (3): 140–144.

Verkhoshansky, Y., and M. Siff. 2009. *Supertraining*. Rome: Ultimate Athletic Concepts.

Vleeming, A., V. Mooney, and R. Stoeckart, eds. 2007. *Movement, Stability and Lumbopelvic Pain: Integration of Research and Therapy*. Edinburgh, UK: Elsevier.

Vleeming A., R. Stoeckart, A. C. W. Volkers, and C. J. Snijders. 1990. "Relation between Form and Function in the Sacroiliac Joint. Part 1: Clinical Anatomical Concepts." *Spine* 15 (2): 130–132.

Vleeming A., A. C. W. Volkers, C. J. Snijders, and R. Stoeckart. 1990. "Relation between Form and Function in the Sacroiliac Joint. Part 2: Biomechanical Aspects." *Spine* 15 (2): 133–136.

Vleeming, A., M. Schuenke, A. Masi, J. Carreiro, L. Danneels, and F. Willard. 2012. "The Sacroiliac Joint: An Overview of its Anatomy, Function and Potential Clinical Implications." *Journal of Anatomy* 221 (6): 537–567.

Vogel, S. 2001. *Prime Mover: A Natural History of Muscle*. New York: W. W. Norton.

Vogel, S., and A. DeFerrari. 2013. *Comparative biomechanics*. Princeton, NJ: Princeton University Press.

Warrener, A., K. Lewton, H. Pontzer, and D. Lieberman. 2015. "A Wider Pelvis Does Not Increase Locomotor Cost in Humans, with Implications for the Evolution of Childbirth." *PLOS ONE* 10 (3): e0118903.

White, T. D., and P. A. Folkens. 2005. *The Human Bone Manual*. Edinburgh, UK: Elsevier.

Whittington, B., A. Silder, B. Heiderscheit, and D. Thelen. 2008. "The Contribution of Passive-Elastic Mechanisms to Lower Extremity Joint Kinetics during Human Walking." *Gait & Posture* 27 (4): 628–634.

Wilke, J., F. Krause, L. Vogt, and W. Banzer. 2016. "What Is Evidence-Based about Myofascial Chains: A Systematic Review." *Archives of Physical Medicine and Rehabilitation* 97 (3): 454–461.

Wrangham, R. 2009. *Catching Fire: How Cooking Made Us Human*. London: Profile Books.

Wynn, T., and F. L. Coolidge. 2012. *How to Think Like a Neandertal*. New York: Oxford University Press.

Yahia, L. H., P. Pigeon, and E. A. DesRosiers. 1993. "Viscoelastic Properties of the Human Lumbodorsal Fascia." *Journal of Biomedical Engineering* 15 (5): 425–429.

Zorn, A. 2007a. "Physical Forms about Structure: The Elasticity of Fascia." *Structural Integration* (March): 15–17.

———. 2007b. "The Swing Walkers of Zambia." *Structural Integration* (December): 20–21.

———. 2015. "Elastic Walking." In Schleip and Baker 2015, 280–296.

Zorn, A., and K. Hodeck. 2011. "Walk with Elastic Fascia: Use the Springs in Your Step!" In Dalton 2011, 96–123.

INDEX

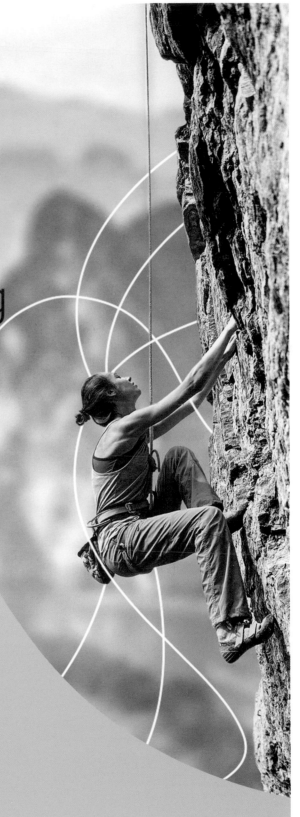

Fascial Release *for* Structural Balance

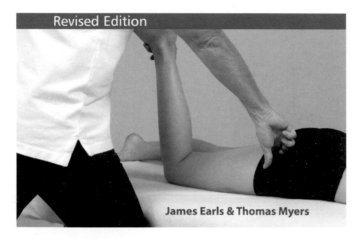

Revised Edition

James Earls & Thomas Myers

This thoroughly revised edition of *Fascial Release for Structural Balance* expands its extensive library of techniques and includes current research on the role and treatment of fascia and myofascia in the body. James Earls and Thomas Myers offer the reader more sophisticated testing to explore the relationship between anatomical structure and function, making this updated edition an essential guide for every practitioner.

Fascia, the biological fabric surrounding muscles, bones, and organs, plays a crucial role in both mobility and stability. By learning to work intelligently with the variety of fascial tissues, a bodyworker can help ease many chronic conditions, often providing immediate and lasting pain relief, as well as reducing the strains that contribute to movement limitations. The authors show that approaching fascial restriction requires "a different eye, a different touch, and tissue-specific techniques."

This book offers a detailed introduction to structural and functional anatomy and fascial release therapy, including "bodyreading"—global postural analysis—coupled with complete technique descriptions. The book features 150 color photographs that clearly demonstrate each technique. Earls and Myers, both respected bodywork professionals, provide any manual therapist— physiotherapists, osteopaths, chiropractors, myofascial trigger point therapists, and massage therapists—the information they need to deliver effective treatments and create systemic change in clients' posture and function.

ISBN 978 1 905367 76 4 (UK); 978 1 623171 00 1 (US) I £24.99/$34.95 I 312 pages I 250 colour illustrations and photographs I paperback